HanGawi Restaurant

a vegetarian shrine in another space and time

Voted top vegetarian restaurant in NYC
- Zagat Survey 2008

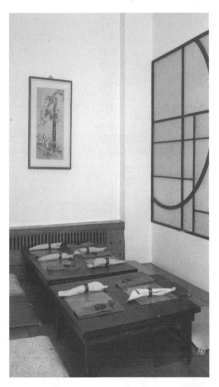

12 East 32nd Street
New York, NY 10016
T.212.213.0077
F.212.689.0780
info@hangawirestaurant.com
www.hangawirestaurant.com

HANGAWI

W9-AXZ-450

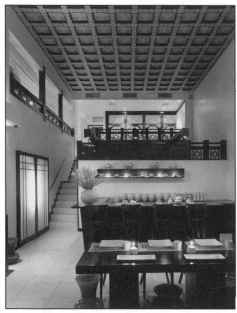
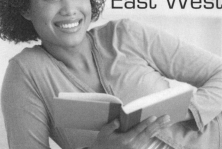

The

Vegan Guide

To

New York City

RYNN BERRY & CHRIS A. SUZUKI

With Barry Litsky, J.D.

Published by

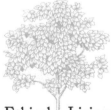

Ethical Living

This book is dedicated to FM Esfandiary, Napoleao Nelson Salgado-Santos, and to all people who respect animals enough not to eat them or consume their byproducts.

•

Fifteenth edition, 2009

ISBN 13: 978-0-9788132-2-2
ISBN 10: 0-9788132-2-7

Library of Congress Number 2001-135857

This book is printed on durable, acid-free paper.

Published in the United States by Ethical Living
P O Box 8174
JAF Station
New York, NY 10116

Cover design and title page design by Donna Hughes and Dr. Chris Abreu-Suzuki. Cover drawing by Sarah Caplan.

Our thanks to Carolyn Handel, Diane Brandt, and J.C. Oliveira.

CONTENTS

Appreciations

"More than a food guide, a portable conscience. "

New York Times

"The Vegan Guide to New York City is a very complete Guide!"

The New York Daily News

"Packed with information and insightful commentary, THE VEGAN GUIDE TO NEW YORK CITY invites you to take a juicy, cholesterol-free, cruelty-free bite out of the Big Apple.

Michael Klaper, M.D.
Author, Vegan Nutrition: Pure and Simple

"Indispensable for the traveling vegan, this guide will most definitely enhance the vegan experience in New York. As a long-time resident of this city, I learned a great deal!"

Gary Francione, Professor of Law, Rutgers University
Director, Animal Rights Law Clinic

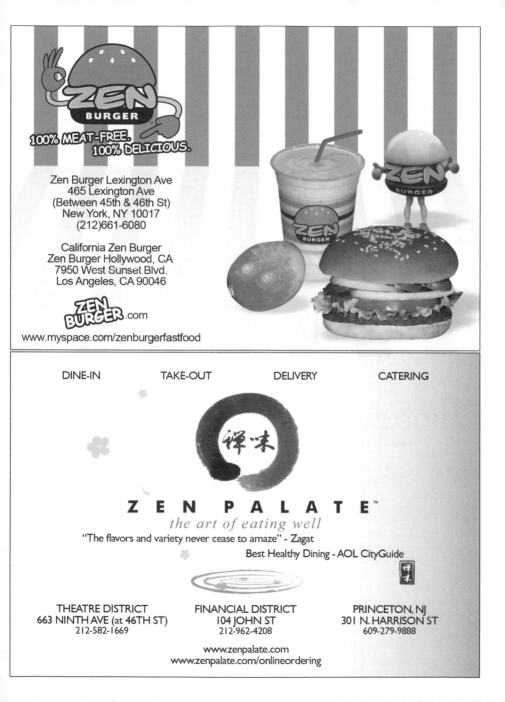

A WORD FROM THE AUTHORS

We love food. Whatever image the uninformed may hold of vegans as joyless ascetics who subsist on carrots and brown rice, it certainly does not hold true for us. We love to eat from a world of varied cuisines—a simple macrobiotic meal of miso soup and steamed vegetables one day, a sumptuous Italian feast of grilled pizza with roasted sweet peppers and portobello mushrooms the next, a rich Thai or Indian curry dinner the third—and one of the joys of New York City is that you can find them all within the same block. That's because New York is a world city.

The Vegan Guide to New York City was launched back in 1994, when Rynn Berry, Max Friedman, and Dan Mills, under the tutelage of Alex Bourke, author of Vegetarian London, put together the first slender edition. That same year Dan went back to London to practice law, and Max went to graduate school to get a Ph.D. in American History. That left Rynn Berry in New York City to carry on with the Vegan Guide. In the years since, Rynn has put out a new edition of the guide annually. In 2001, he joined forces with Chris Abreu Suzuki, and Barry Litsky to put out the first quality paperback edition of the Vegan Guide. Rynn, Chris and Barry met at the Farm Sanctuary, a refuge for farm animals in Watkins Glen, New York.

Rynn Berry is the historical advisor to the North American Vegetarian Society. He is the author of several seminal books on vegetarianism; they include *The New Vegetarians, Famous Vegetarians and Their Favorite Recipes, Hitler: Neither Vegetarian Nor Animal Lover, and Food for The Gods Vegetarianism and the World's Religions.* In 2004, Rynn was commissioned to write a 6,000 word entry on the history of vegetarianism in the US for the *Oxford Encyclopedia of Food and Drink in America.* In 2007, he had seven entries published in the *Oxford Companion to American Food and Drink.* In 2008, he was the guest expert on the vegan lifestyle in New York City for The New Yotk Times City Room Blog. Rynn contributes frequently to both scholarly and spiritual publications.

Chris Abreu-Suzuki, Ph.D., is a professor of Mathematics, a long distance runner, who has won many races, a fervent animal rights activist and a connoisseur of vegan food. She's been a vegan since 1992 and an ethical vegetarian since 1977.

Barry Litsky, an intellectual property lawyer, who lives in New York City, does pro bono work for animal rights causes. He is also a vegetarian gourmet, who loves to whip up vegan meals for friends in his apartment.

Some Of Our Guests Come To Heal. Some Come To Learn...

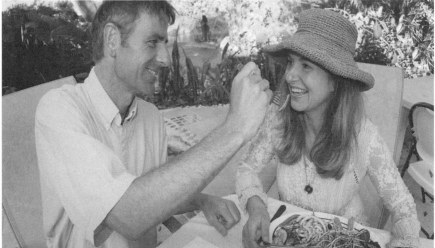

...Others Come Simply For The Food.

We really don't believe it matters what brings you here, because once you arrive, you'll realize that you're going to receive all of the above and more. You cannot help but to heal in the atmosphere that we've created and with lectures and classes going on all day long, you're sure to learn more than you thought possible. But the World-Class Raw Cuisine will definitely be at the top of the list of things that make your Hippocrates experience a memorable one.

• Delicious Organic Living Foods • Life Changing Lectures • Wheatgrass & Juice Therapies • Medical & Dark Field Analysis • Ozonated Pools, Saunas & Spas • Exercise Classes - Group & Individual • Yoga, Meditation & Qigong • Skilled Professional Massage Therapists • Hyperbaric Therapies • Diapulse • Immune System Building IV Therapies • Oxygen Therapy Procedures • Aqua Chi • Psychological Counseling & Mind Mastery • Electromagnetic, Turbosonic & Vibrosaun • Medical & Nutritional Counseling • Store & Gift Shop with Books, Music & DVD's
+ A Complete Line of Organic Supplements
+ Organic Essential Oils and Make Up

Call today for a free brochure and DVD, toll-free 1-800-842-2125 or visit us on the web - www.hippocratesinstitute.org

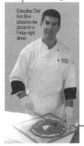

Executive Chef Ken Blue preparing raw pizzas for a Friday night dinner.

HIPP CRATES
HEALTH INSTITUTE
1443 Palmdale Court • West Palm Beach, Florida
561-471-8876

A FEW NOTES ON DINING IN NEW YORK...

There are more than 100 restaurants described in this book, but by no means should you limit yourself to them. New York is a city where you have the wide world at your doorstep, and you should not hesitate to plunge right in. All the restaurants listed in this guide offer vegan meals, but vegans will also do well at restaurants that do not go out of their way to cater to them, bearing in mind a few basic principles.

There are two centers for Indian food in town. One is 6th Street between 1st and 2nd Avenues, a block known as "Little India" for its cheek-by-jowl Indian restaurants. The joke is that there's one kitchen and a conveyor belt. Less well known to tourists is the community on Lexington around 28th Street, where the patrons are often Indian, too. As a rule, you should ask if they cook with ghee (clarified butter). We've listed Indian restaurants that use oil in most of their dishes, but ask anyway. You can request that they leave off the raita (yogurt with cucumbers).

There has been a boom in the popularity of Mexican food in the United States in the past few years, notably when salsa bypassed ketchup in condiment sales. In Mexico, Mexican food is based on corn or wheat with beans, but prepared with lard, cheese and meat stock, making strict vegan travel there a challenge. In New York City, there are a few authentic and many cheap Americanized places to eat Mexican food unsuitable for vegans. However, the last five years has seen an explosion in the number of trendy, "Cal-Mex" or "Tex-Mex" or "San Francisco Style" restaurants serving a healthy variation of Mexican cuisine prepared without lard, containing fresh vegetables and usually with the option of soy cheese, whole wheat tortillas and brown rice. (Almost all soy cheeses contain casein, a milk derivative; most tofu sour cream does not. See Glossary.) We have included addresses for these chains of healthy, vegan-friendly Mexican restaurants, where some of the best meals in the city are to be had. While they are similar, we give Burritoville a slight edge over the others:

Some of the most talented chefs in town are at moderate to expensive Italian restaurants. Vegans can always find something to eat here, if you request that your food be prepared with olive oil instead of butter, and make sure they leave out the common flavorings of Parmesan cheese and prosciutto (ham). Fresh pasta is often, but not always, made with egg. At Thai restaurants, it's dried shrimp and fish sauce you want to look out for. But we should offer this caveat: Since non-veg restaurants use utensils and working surfaces that may have come in contact with animal flesh, it is always preferable to eat in vegetarian/ vegan restaurants to avoid cross-contamination. Now go ahead and explore.

Nearly every restaurant in this guide offers take-out (meals to take home) and almost all of them also will deliver food right to your door, if you're in the area (say, within fifteen to twenty blocks). Because this service is nearly universal, we have specified only when a restaurant does NOT deliver or serve take-out. Otherwise, if the weather's bad or you'd rather stay indoors, you can call any one of these places and have your dinner in the comfort of your own room. Delivery is almost always free, usually with a minimum total order of $7-12, and you should tip your delivery person 15% of the bill. You can simply call up and tell them what you want, or ask what they have without meat or milk products; or, better still, do as New Yorkers do and start

your own collection of take-out menus from your favorite restaurants .

Most health food shops offer an assortment of ready
eat foods for vegans—hummus sandwiches, nutburgers and salads—in the refrigerator case.
These tend to be OK, range in price from two to four dollars and can be just the thing if you want
a quick snack. We've made a note by health food shops that go a little further, with a fresh salad
bar, sandwich counter or buffet.

More and more liquor stores in New York stock organic wines, and of these, several labels are
vegan—they use no fish or eggs in the "fining" (clarifying) process. Look for anything by the
Organic Wine Works label or anything by Frey except the 1991 Cabernet, which was fined with
egg whites. If you can't find them anywhere, try Warehouse Wines and Spirits at 735 Broadway
(at Astor Place) or the slightly more expensive Astor Wines and Spirits at Lafayette and Astor.

An important note for our foreign readers: tax and tip are NOT included in the price at American
restaurants, so figure on adding another 8.65% for the city and 15
20% for the service. American servers get paid an abysmal hourly wage and earn most of their
salary from tips, so this is not really optional: unless you get terrible service, everyone leaves
15% as a matter of routine, and it's nicer to leave 20%. An exception is when there is no server,
as in buffets or self
serve cafeterias; and when you dine in a group of more than five persons, the tip ("gratuity") may
be figured into your total. People who deliver take-out to your door should also get a 15% tip.

A valid current Student I.D. will get you 10-15% off at many restaurants and some shops. The
restaurants are grouped by neighborhood, and listed alphabetically within each neighborhood.

A NOTE ON OUR POLICY OF RESTAURANT SELECTION:

In 1994, when we first launched this guide, the number of vegan and vegetarian restaurants were
rather sparse; so we included some vegetarian friendly restaurants that served some meat, but
went out of their way to accommodate vegetarians. As of 1996, it was our feeling that we should
no longer include any restaurants that served animal flesh of any kind--be it fish or fowl, snail or
cow--because all restaurants have become friendlier to vegetarians; so to continue to feature
vegetarian friendly restaurants in the Guide would make it meaningless. The vegetarian friendly
restaurants that were included in the original guide were grandfathered in and phased out as they
closed. In a few instances, restaurants started out as being vegan, then started serving increasing
amounts of meat. These were so egregiously non-veg. that we had to delete them from the guide.
But from then on, only vegetarian and vegan restaurants were to be included. That's why you
may not find the trendy almost-vegetarian restaurant that you've been hearing about. Look to the
conventional guides for those. Furthermore, in rating and ranking restaurants, we add and
subtract points depending on how vegan they are. In other words, if they use honey or dairy
products in their dishes, they will be penalized for it.

THE RESTAURANTS

HARLEM
(North of Central Park)

CAFE VEG [ve] **$**

Full service
West Indian
No cards
No alcohol

2291 Seventh Avenue
brt/ 134th/135th Streets
212-491-3223
M-Su 11am-9pm

The rasta chefs at Veggie Castle in Brooklyn, and the Uptown Juice Bar in Harlem, were the first in the city to serve tasty vegan fast food with a Caribbean fillip. So it's great to see that Veggie Castle has just opened a branch in Queens, and that the Uptown Juice Bar has just opened this sister restaurant on 135th Street. We swilled the Mock BBQ Chicken Wrap served with Goddess

Dressing, plus three sides--Okra, Collard Greens and Mashed Potatoes in just a few minutes. Then we slurped their tonic juices. The sharp-eyed waitress looked at us a touch disapprovingly, we thought, as we tottered out the door. True: we had eaten with unseemly gusto. But that's how we behave when we're around delicious Ital food.But wait, isn't that a pleonasm?

HEIGHTS VEGETARIAN [ve]$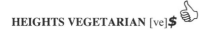

	1121 St. Nicholas Avenue
Counter service	at 166th Street (Washington Heights)
Vegan Ital food	718-927-0908
All cards	daily 8am-8pm
No alcohol	

Concert promoter Morton Hall, who has promoted concerts for legendary performers James Brown, Miles Davis , and Stevie Wonder, has partnered with David Simmons--the owner of Café Veg, and the Uptown Juice Bar-- to found a new Ital Eatery on West 166th Street called Heights Vegetarian. It serves the same delicious Ital food familiar to those who've eaten at Café Veg. or Uptown Juice bar, but it does so in a sleek setting hard by the Columbia Medical Center, whose physicians and nurses make up the preponderance of the restaurant's clientele.

We sampled the eats with our friend George Guimaraes who opened the first vegan restaurant in South America--Vegethus at Villa Mariana in Sao Paulo, Brazil. George had never tasted Ital food, and was besotted with it. So, it was love at first bite! We sampled their Phlouri, a fritter made with split pea flour and turmeric. This we followed with a combination plate containing a spicy Lasagna, Soy Terriyaki Chunks, Pumpkin and Collard Greens. We chased it with a Cleansing Cocktail a combination of carrot apple and beet juice blended with ginger. For dessert, we had the Carrot Cake and a Death By Chocolate that left us with a decided *rictus mortis*.

Mr. Hall started Heights vegetarian to give his daughters a business to run. From the high quality of the food and from the obvious fact that vegan restaurants are a growth industry, we would say he made a sound investment.

RAW SOUL [ve] $$

	348 West 145th Street
Counter service	bet. St. Nicholas/ Edgecomb
Organic juice bar & deli	
Avenues	
No cards	212-491-4263
No alcohol	M-Sa 9am-9pm
www.rawsoul@rawsoul.com	Su 11am-4pm

This is the real soul food--not the ham hocks and fat backs that the plantation owners forced on the slaves. The real soul food was the living- foods diet of fruits and vegetables that the African peoples lived on before so many of them were transported in chains to the New World. Eddie and Lillian Robinson, husband and wife partners, have helped to revive the tradition of eating

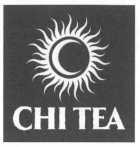
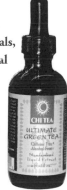

healthy and delicious unfired foods in the black community. Theirs is some of the tastiest and most affordable living food in town.

By profession, this talented duo are tap dancers; Lillian is also a jazz singer with a CD to her credit. All their artistic talent, and, as they like to emphasize, "love" go into the making of their mouthwatering living vegan food. Vegan is the operative word here. Eddie and Lillian stress that they go out of their way to avoid using dairy products. They serve their home-made almond and sesame milks instead; and they use dates, and agave (cactus) nectar in lieu of honey.

When we arrived, Lillian and Eddie regaled us with a raw Curried Almond-Zucchini Soup that was out of this world. Then they served us a raw Middle Eastern plate consisting of raw Hummus, Tabbouleh and living Falafel Balls made from fava beans. For dessert, Eddie served us a scrumptious living Pear Tart made with macadamia nuts, walnuts, almonds, cashew-cream sauce, and Turkish figs. Need we say m-m-m-m-m-m?

As we were leaving, we remembered that we were planning a picnic on the morrow; so we took home with us a couple of Egyptian Wraps, which consisted of a marinated mixture of zucchini, eggplant, yellow squash and vidalia onions, wrapped in a collard green leaf. We also took along a few bottles each of their live home-made Sorrel Punch, containing hibiscus, wheat berries, dates, raisins, star anise and lime, and their home-made living Ginger Beer, containing rejuvelac, dates, raisins, ginger, cinnamon, and lime.

In 2007, Ras Dawitt, the chef-owner of the popular, but short-lived raw vegan juice bar, Earthly Juices, joined the staff at Raw Soul. At about the same time, Raw Soul moved around the corner into larger quarters to accommodate their growing clientele. Their new space is at street level. Inside, the walls are hung with paintings by local African-American artists on loan from the nearby Simmons gallery. Amidst these vibrant paintings, and the warm ambiance, you may sip the juices and smoothies from the juice bar and savor dishes from the raw deli such as the Rasta Pasta, the Barbecue Burger, The Collard Wrap the Personal Pizza and The Tamale Pie. Eating lustily of these left us deeply satisfied, but still craving more. The desserts run the gamut from raw cakes, cheesecakes, and pies to an array of ice-creams. All their menu items have such robust flavors that you'll probably want to learn how to duplicate them at home. If so, Lillian offers instruction in a series of hands-on courses.

STRICTLY ROOTS |ve| $$

Counter service
West Indian
No cards
No alcohol

2058 Adam Clayton Powell Blvd.
at 123rd Street
212-864-8699
M-Sa 12pm-11pm
Su 12pm-10pm

As the Rasta chef says, there is nothing served here that "crawls, walks, swims or flies." The menu changes every day and consists of items like broccoli & tofu, chick pea stew, seitan, falafel, tofu tempura, or veggie duck. The daily staples include millet, brown rice, greens and fried plantains. You can order small, medium or large portions of any combination of the above for $5, $7.50 and $10 respectively. Don't expect gourmet presentation, but it's good, wholesome stuff. They also have a variety of smaller dishes (e.g. veggie burger, vegetable salad) and beverages—juices, soy milk, and non-alcoholic ginger beer.

![A compassionate world begins with you.]

A compassionate world begins with you.

Since 1986 Farm Sanctuary, the nation's leading farm animal protection organization, has worked to end cruelty to farm animals and promote compassionate living. Farm Sanctuary rescues animals from abject cruelty, exposes the callousness and disregard for life that drive the "food animal" industry, and advocates for legal protections for farm animals. Help us protect the most vulnerable among us, and raise your voice in compassion for farm animals everywhere. To learn more about our shelters, campaigns and educational programs visit www.farmsanctuary.org.

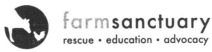

farmsanctuary
rescue · education · advocacy

National Office · P.O. Box 150 · Watkins Glen, NY 14891 · 607-583-2225
www.farmsanctuary.org

UPTOWN JUICE BAR[ve] $

Counter service
West Indian
No cards
No alcohol
www.uptownjuicebar.com

54 West 125th Street
bet. 5th & Lenox
212-289-9501
daily 8am-10pm

A cross between a small cafe and a juice bar, Uptown Juice Bar is to be prized as much for its food as for its juices. Along with an array of juice combinations and smoothies, it serves delicious Caribbean-style vegan food. And although the menu contains alarming words like beef and fish, these are to be understood as "mock beef" and "mock fish." For instance there is a "turkey" salad, a "chicken" salad and a "fish" salad, but no turkey, chicken or fish died to produce these dishes. They're entirely ersatz and are very tasty. We had one of their combination meals that consisted of collard greens, tofu with black mushrooms, and a vegan shepherd's pie. To wash down this delectable grub, have one of their fruit smoothies or a juice tonic that is designed to cure whatever ails you. For impotence, drink a potent brew of carrot, parsley, cucumber, orange, and papaya juices. For asthma, gulp down a beverage containing carrot, celery, and grapefruit juice. Of course, if you're a vegan of long-standing, you probably don't have any of these ailments, so toast your good health--and your good fortune in being a vegan-- with a fruit smoothie instead.

   Indicates we especially recommend this restaurant for the quality of the food.

UPPER WEST SIDE
(West 59th Street and Above)

AYURVEDA CAFE [v] **$$**

Full service	706 Amsterdam Avenue
South Indian	at 94th Street
All cards	212-932-2400
No alcohol	daily 11:30am-11:30pm

With its mango-hued walls and mottled sky blue ceilings, the Ayurveda Cafe resembles nothing so much as a film set for an early Merchant-Ivory movie, like Shakespeare Wallah or Bombay Talkie. So, it's not surprising to learn that the owner, Tirlok Malik, is a film director, who has parlayed a side interest in Indian cuisine into what seems to my taste buds to be one of the best Indian restaurants in town. Part Ismail Merchant, part Deepak Chopra with the Chopra ascendant, Malik has based his restaurant's dishes on the teachings of one of the four sacred books of Vedic Hinduism, which dates back at least 3,000 years--the Ayurveda (which means "knowledge of life" in Sanskrit.) Essentially, Ayurvedic cuisine tries to combine the six tastes, sweet. sour, salty, astringent, bitter and pungent, in order to produce a cuisine that is properly balanced for your body type. It certainly was right for my olfactory type. The Thali that I tasted was lightly spiced and lightly cooked so that you could taste each vegetable. I had to skip the raitas and desserts because they all contained dairy products and /or honey. Otherwise, a vegan can dine very handsomely here.

BLOSSOM[CAFÉ [ve] **$$$** 👍

	466 Columbus Avenue
Full Service	bet. 82nd/ 83rd Streets
Global vegan, orgainc	212-875-2600
All cards	daily 11:30am-10:30pm
Orgainc beer & wine	
www.blossomnyc.com	

See description under Midtown West

CAFE VIVA [A.K.A. VIVA HERBAL PIZZERIA [v] $ 👍

Counter service
Italian vegetarian, kosher
All cards
No alcohol

2578 Broadway
bet.97th//98th Streets
212-663-8482
daily 11am-11pm

The founder, Tony Iracani, tells us that Cafe Viva is the only Italian vegetarian restaurant in the US, which after sampling the vegetarian antipasto and the tasty cheeseless pizzas, strikes us as shameful. Italian restaurateurs should beat a path to Cafe Viva to see how vegan Italian food is done, then go forth and do likewise. We had the Pizza Pura, a dairy-free, yeast-free spelt crust, topped with tofu marinated in Miso, grilled veggies and spinach with a vegetarian antipasto on the side. The fridge is stocked with healthful sodas such as Twisted Bean Vanilla Brew, Borealis Birch Beer, Ginseng tonics and China Cola. Recently Cafe Viva has expanded its menu to include a super anti-oxidant pizza; a Zen pizza, which features a green-tea herbal crust; tofu marinated with herbs, and a green tea pesto; it is topped off with a layer of maitake and shitake mushrooms. Another favorite is the Santa Rosa, which consists of a whole wheat crust layered with tofu marinated in miso, and topped off with sun-dried tomatoes and roasted garlic. Viva offers two types of vegan Lasagna as well as vegan Calzones made from spelt and whole wheat. Other pastas such as Raviolis, Strombolis, and Zitis are made from scratch and can be veganized to order. The service staff is friendly and helpful to the point of being obsequious. One of the great pleasures apart from the food is that one can sit and read a paper or chat with a companion for hours without being hurried or pressured. We say, "Viva! Cafe Viva!"

HUMMUS PLACE [v]$

Full Service
Kosher Israeli hummus house
All cards
Wine & Beer

305 Amstardam Avenue
bet. W. 74th/ W. 75th Streets
212-799-3335
M-Su 10am-12am

See description under Greenwich Village and other location under East Village.

MAOZ [v] $

Counter service
Israeli falafel shack, kosher
All Cards
No alcohol
www.maozusa.com

2047 A Broadway
bet. 70th/ 71st Streets
212-362-2622
daily 11am-12am

See description under Midtown East and other location under East Village.

19

UPPER EAST SIDE
(East 59th Street and Above)

CANDLE CAFE [ve]**$$$** 👍

1307 Third Avenue
Full service   bet. 74th/75th Streets
Vegan, organic   212-472-0970 & 472-7169(fax)
All cards   M-Sa 11:30am-10:30pm
Organic wine and beer   Su 11:30am-9:30pm
www. candlecafe.com

Back in the days when Bart Potenza, Candle's tousle-haired founder, ran a juice bar called the Healthy Candle, he dreamed of owning a vegan restaurant. A few years later, he realized his dream when he opened Candle Cafe. *Fourteen years later,* Candle Cafe has metamorphosed into one of New York's most popular eateries where celebrity watchers can spot environmental- and health-conscious actors like Woody Harrelson, and Alicia Silverstone, or prominent Animal Rights activists like Eddy Lama of The Witness , or Harold Brown of The Peaceable Kingdom.

They come here because Bart and his partner, Joy Pierson, have a history of supporting environmental and animal rights causes and because they serve up some of the tastiest vegan food in town. We found just about everything on the menu appetizing, but our particular favorites were as follows: Our favorite appetizer was the Seitan Chimichurri (South American marinated seitan skewers with creamy citrus *herb sauce.)* Our favorite entree was the Cabernet-Infused Seitan *(pan-seared seitan* served with steamed greens and coleslaw). We also relished the Tuscan Lasagna with Grilled Summer Vegetables, Tofu-Basil Ricotta, and Seitan Ragout with a Truffled Tomato Sauce. For dessert, we fell upon the Chocolate Mousse Pie and the Decadent Chocolate Cake with Vanilla Frosting. When it comes to Seitan dishes, which are the forte of both Candle Cafe and Candle 79, no other restaurant can hold a candle to the Candle.

CANDLE 79 [ve] **$$$** 👍

154 East 79th Street
Full service   at Lexington Avenue
Global organic vegan   212-537-7179
All cards   M-Sa Lunch, 12pn-3:30pm
Organic wines, beers and sakes.   Dinner, 5:30pm-10:30pm
                         Su   Brunch, 12pm-4pm
                              Dinner, 5-10pm

A special gluten-free menu is available. Private party rooms are also available.

Now at last New York's Upper East Side has a posh vegan restaurant serving Global Organic style vegan cuisine that can rival --in elegance as well as in sapidity- Millennium in San Francisco, Chu Chai in Montreal, Vegethus in Sao Paulo, Bann's Vegetarian Cafe in Edinburgh and Hangawi in midtown New York.

Bart Potenza and his partner Joy Pierson have transformed an unprepossessing two-story town house that was formerly a prosaic restaurant called the Dining Room into a restaurant whose interior design is as ravishing as are the dishes on its bill of fare. Start with a glass of organic Sangria at the intimate downstairs wine and sake bar. With an extensive all-organic wine and sake cocktail list, Candle 79's sleek and sexy bar is a popular spot for eco-chic dates!

At the table, begin with the Teaser: delicious stuffed manicotti with sautéed mushrooms, tofu-basil cheese, seitan ragout, toasted cashew parmesan cheese, roasted tomato sauce and pine nut pesto.

Then proceed to the Wild Mushroom Salad with Arugala, Grape Tomatoes, Roasted Cippolini Onions, and Creamy Horseradish Dressing. Then on to the maincourse of Grilled Balsamic Seitan with grilled corn and shallots, fingerling potato chips, sautéed green beans, and peach salsa. If you are a rawfoodist, try the wonderfully flavorful Live Zucchini Enchiladas. Finish with the ever-addictive Chocolate-Peanut Butter Bliss- a creamy mousse confection nestled in a dark chocolate shell. Be sure to check the current menu on-line (www. candlecafe.com), as it changes with the season according to local organic produce. Much of the credit for Candle 79's dazzling menu is owing to head chef Angel Ramos, and pastry chef Jorge Pineda. We are avid fans of their seitan dishes both at Candle Cafe and at Candle 79. They have raised the preparation of Seitan to high art. Indeed, their Seitan Piccata (Sir Paul McCartney's favorite!)with Creamed Spinach, Savory Potato Cake and Lemon-Caper Sauce should make Seitan worshippers of even the most fundamentalist carnivore. Congratulations to Candle 79 for being named "Best Vegetarian Restaurant " in Zagat's 2007 and 2008!

GOBO [ve] **$$** 👍

Full service
Organic, Asian-Western fusion cuisine
All cards
Organic beer & wine
www.goborestaurant.com

1426 Third Avenue
at 81st Street
212-288-4686
Su-We 11:30am-11:30pm
Th-Sa 11:30am-12am

See the description under East Village.

GREEN BEAN, THE [v] **$** 👍

1413 York Avenue
Counter service
bet. 75th/ 76th Streets
Homestyle organic vegetarian
212-861-8060
Visa & Mastercard
daily 8am-9pm
No alcohol
www. BeanGoneGreen.com

When we walked into the Green Bean, shortly after it opened, we saw three generations of the owner's family all of whom were vegetarian, all working behind the counter. There's Darrel the owner, Darrel's mother, Barbara, and Darrel's nephew, Nirmal. Darrel also owns the restaurant down the block called Beanochio. In fact, the Green Bean now occupies the space formerly inhabited by Beanocchio, which outgrew its space. That's what beans do; they grow and grow as if by magic.

As we know from *Jack and the Beanstalk,* beans have magical properties. And this Green Bean is no exception. Magical is it that such a small space can produce such a high volume of high quality dishes and beverages.

Appropriately enough we started with a beany dish--their Spicy Tempeh with Mixed Greens and Sweet Potatoes. Superb! Next we tried their Seitan Cutlets with Mashed Potatoes and Miso Gravy. Pluperfect!

Their smoothies are made with organic frozen fruit and contain no added ice. (Most juice bars spike their fruit with superadded ice as a stretcher.) We quaffed the Berry Smoothie, and ii really socked our knocks off!

For dessert we munched cookies and cupcakes, which are all vegan, all delicious, and all baked downstairs in the basement. Needless to say, we left feeling satisfied and full of beans, magic beans

PONGAL [v] **$$**

1154 First Avnue
Full service
at 63rd Street
Indian vegetarian
212-355-4600
All majjor cards
Th 11:30am-10pm
No alcohol
F-Su 11:30am-10:30pm

See the description under Midtown East.

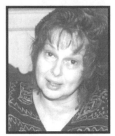
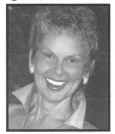
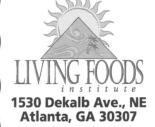

MIDTOWN WEST and Chelsea
(West 14th to West 59th Streets)

BLOSSOM [ve] $$$

Full Service
Global vegan, orgainc
All cards
Orgainc beer & wine
www.blossomnyc.com

187 Ninth Avenue
bet. 21st/ 22nd Streets
212-627-1144
daily 11:30am-10:30pm

Erstwhile actors, Ronen Seri, and his wife Pamela, couldn't find a restaurant to satisfy their recherché vegan tastes; so they decided to open their own place. We vegan foodies are all in their debt. For now we have someplace to go besides Candle '79, on the upper east side, and Millennium, in San Francisco, to slake our appetite for organic vegan haute cuisine.

Indeed the restaurant's interior has a touch of the theater about it. With its chic townhouse setting; its cozy fireplace; its burnished wood tables; its floor-to-ceiling draperies; it looks like the perfect stage set for a posh restaurant

Despite their restaurant's high-toned elegance, Ronen and Pamela are not above stating, right on their menu, that "Blossom is first and foremost animal caring." Consequently, their "food is not only organic, it is also dairy and cholesterol free." This is the first time we know of that a restaurateur has had the courage to remind his/her patrons that conventional non-veg. food involves the wanton sacrifice of our fellow creatures.

We would eat at Blossom out of solidarity with Ronen and Pamela--just to pay tribute to their ethical approach to food preparation--but, fortunately, their food is so extraordinary that we also eat there for the sheer yumminess of the dishes.

Everyone we know. in our circle of vegan friends , raves about Blossom's appetizers--especially the South Asian Lumpia (curried seitan and potatoes wrapped in a crispy chickpea crepe, served with mango onion sambal). And, we are here to confirm that it, and the Black-Eyed Pea Cake (crispy cake of yukon gold potato & black-eyed peas, served with chipotle aioli) are as fresh and peppery as they're cracked up to be.

We're confessed seitan worshippers; so we reveled in the Barbecued Seitan Sandwich (barbecued seitan and caramelized onions with fresh cut fries or salad); and the Seitan Medallions (pan seared seitan cutlets served with herbed soft polenta and broccoli rabe). They would have delighted Old Split-foot himself, [who like most ungulates is doubtless a vegan].

For dessert we had the Chocolate Ganache Cake (a layered combination of rich chocolate ganache and chocolate cake). And the Pineapple Crepe (grilled pineapple wrapped in a crepe served with coconut reduction and green tea or vanilla ice-cream). It was a fitting climax to this play in three courses. We were chagrined--as with most extraordinary theater--only that it had to end.

DALE & THOMAS POPCORN [v] $

Counter-service
Indiana popcorn
All Major cards
No alcohol

1592 Broadway
at 48th Street
212-581-1872
M-Sa 11am-11pm
Su 11am-12am

This is one of those single-food-item eateries--like Hummus Place, Pommes Frites, Cafe Viva Pizzeria, Moshe's Falafel and the Dosa Hut--in which New York abounds. If one can make a meal of Pommes Frites, then why not dine on popcorn that is freshly popped on the spot? Select from an array of flavors-- Back-Yard Barbecue, Drive-In, Kettle Corn, Caramel, Chocolate Chunk On Caramel, Dark and White Chocolate, etc. If you're a vegan, you'll want to eschew the Cheddar and the Chocolate, which are made with cheese and milk-powder respectively, but the others are blessedly dairy-free.[Canola oil is used instead of butter].Munch them on the spot, smuggle them into your favorite Bijou, or take them home and snack on them while watching the Purple Rose of Cairo on your DVD player.

See other location under Upper West Side.

DESI JUNCTION [v] $

Counter service
Punjabi homestyle
All Cards
No alcohol

688 10th Avenue
bet. 48th/ 49th Streets
212-956-0185
M-Sa 9:30am-12:30am
Su 1pm-1am

The name of this restaurant sounds like a Bollywood action movie, and the walls are festooned with portraits of Indian film stars, but the food here outshines the most effulgent Bollywood stars. The chef who presides over this celestial banquet, Vipur, hails from Delhi. She is a vegetarian from birth, having been raised according to the strictest dietary precepts of Hinduism, which prohibit the eating of animal flesh. We've found that some of the best Indian veg. chefs in the city are women, and chef Vipur's ' food would seem to bear out this thesis. She does things with tofu and soy foods that we've never encountered in an Indian restaurant. For some reason, most Indian veg. chefs seem to be stymied by tofu, Vipur, happily, is not! We were particularly smitten with her Tofu Delight (bean curd stir-fried with onions and tomatoes, bell pepper and sauteed with spices); her Matar Mushroom Tofu (peas and mushrooms tofu cooked in a thick authentic curry); her Special Soyabean (A high protein delicacy made with chunks of shredded soyabean in an exotic thick curry with peas.)

She will custom cook for each diner, which is great for vegans, who don't want their dishes tainted with liquid meat or dairy products.[No ghee is used in any of the dishes.] Each dish will be adjusted to the degree of spiciness and heat that one desires.

Her business partner, Hardip Singh, is a Sikh. Like most traditional Sikhs he is a vegetarian from birth. He told us, by the by, that a disproportionate number of cab drivers in NYC are vegetarian Sikhs. Why? we wondered. He couldn't really say. Perhaps its due to their entrepreneurial spirit, or their innate derring-do?

The food is budget priced. In fact Desi Junction offers the cheapest buffet in Manhattan--$4.99 for a bowl of rice and two veg. Even cheaper is the special, which entitles you to a bowl of rice and one veg. dish for $3.. And the food is so authentic that it attracts Sikh cab drives from all five boroughs In fact you may have to fight for a table with the Sikh cabby who drove you to the Junction.

DIMPLE [v] $

Self-service
Indian, kosher
All major cards
No alcohol

11 West 30th Street
bet. Fifth Avenue/Broadway
212-643-9464
M-F 8:30am-10pm
Sa, Su 11am-10pm

This fast-food Indian vegetarian restaurant will put dimples in the cheeks of famished midtown office workers who at lunch time are hard put to find a good vegetarian restaurant in the vicinity. Not only is the food good here, but it's so economical as to make the budget-conscious vegetarian consider eating here rather than brown-bagging it. The cost of a take-out Thali that includes a choice of three vegetables, dal or kadhi, rice, 2 roti or one naan, or 2 pakoras, raita, pickle, salad and a sweet is only $5.99. Each day they offer a different Thali from a different region of India: Monday it's a Gujarati Thali; Thursday, it's a Sindhi Thali. The only caveat is that vegans must be careful to ask which dishes contain dairy products and which do not.

See other location in Queens.

FRUIT SALADS, FRUIT SHAKES [ve] $

Food cart
Fruit salads and shakes
All cards
No alcohol

Corner 46th Street
at Sixth Avenue
(no phone)
M-F 7am-4pm

Just as we had opined in our review of New York Dosas--that one of New York's finest vegan restaurants is actually a food cart--so we must assert that one of New York's best rawfood restaurants and juice bars is really a food cart. The cart is owned by a jaunty middle-aged Vietnamese couple named Vo and Do An. Their fruit salads and shakes are ambrosial. The salads, which range in price from $2.50-$3.50, can be made to order in any combination of fruits and vegetables such as mango, pears, lettuce and carrots. There is a wide array of fruits to choose from--papayas, cherries, blueberries, strawberries, cantaloupes, etc.

The shakes, which range in price from $3.00 for a small to $4.00 for a large, are so generous as to be a meal in themselves. Choose from such combinations as mango, banana and pineapple, and strawberry, mango and banana. There are ten possible combinations to select from.

The eating of animal flesh extinguishes the great seed of compassion

THE BUDDHA (SIDDHARTHA GAUTAMA OR SHAKYAMUNI)
563 BC-483 BC from *The Mahaparinirvana*

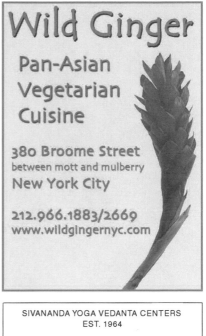
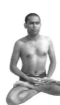

all creatures great and small

Millions of Americans love animals. But many creatures still suffer from cruel and abusive treatment.

Help us confront animal cruelty in all its forms. Visit **humanesociety.org** to find out what you can do.

Celebrating Animals | Confronting Cruelty

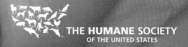

THE **HUMANE** SOCIETY
OF THE UNITED STATES

The word "shake" has the connotation in North America of a beverage that combines fruit, ice-cream and milk, but no dairy products are used here. Vo and Do An are from a Buddhist country in which dairy products have traditionally been eschewed on moral grounds. [Eating dairy products like meat-eating is a violation of the first precept of Buddhism, *ahimsa:* "Non-violence to all living creatures."] Consequently, Do An and Vo do not put milk or yogurt in the fruit shakes. or salads. The shakes and salads are composed purely of fruit. Nor do any of their shakes or salads contain frozen fruit or fruit syrups made from concentrate, as do those of most of the juice bars in the city.

Do An and Vo work year round, sleet or snow, rain or shine. But when one drinks their shakes, or eats one of their fruit salads, it always feels like a sun-splashed day in midsummer!

MOSHE'S FALAFEL[ve] $ 👍

	Corner 46th Street
Food cart	at Sixth Avenue
Middle Eastern (Israeli), kosher	(no phone)
No cards	M-Th 11am-5pm
No alcohol	F 11am-3pm

Let's face it: most falafel places in the city are just plain "foul-awful!" Mainly, we think, this is because of the cross-contamination. All-too-often, the "foul-awfuls" in non-veg. places are deep-fried in the same rancid oil that is used to cook animal flesh. At this outdoor food cart, however--because the food is vegan and kosher--none of these concerns apply.

Perhaps it was psychological, but knowing that the falafels weren't contaminated made them taste that much better. Evidently, Moshe's customers concur, because when we sampled his food, there was a line around the block! Portions are generous. Topped with colossal pickles, stuffed with chunks of tomato, fistfuls of lettuce, and drenched with the obligatory tahini sauce, Moshe's Falafels are fully twice the size of the standard-issue falafel sandwich. For those who like their falafels hot, ask for a devilishly piquant hot sauce on the side. Or if you're traveling any distance before eating it, ask for the tahini sauce on the side too. [The trick to eating a falafel sandwich is to eat it on the spot lest the tahini sauce seep into the bread and make it soggy. And nothing tastes worse than a soggy falafel sandwich!] Moshe serves up an ample salad and a selection of vegan soups as well.

NATURAL GOURMET COOKERY SCHOOL [ve] $$$ 👍

	48 West 21st Street
Full service	bet 5th and 6th Avenues
Gourmet vegan	212-645-5170
All cards	F 6:30pm
BYOB	

Every Friday, the Natural Gourmet Cookery School has a feast that is prepared by the students at the school. The public is invited to partake of the students' cooking, which is vegan. Students, attired as waiters, serve four-course meals at large communal dining tables that are reminiscent of a college refectory. As in a college dining hall, the communal tables encourage the dinner guests to strike up conversations with total strangers, which adds to the convivial atmosphere.

The price for the four-course meal, at thirty-two dollars, is high, but then the cooking rivals that of any four-star restaurant. Truth to tell, we did overhear a few diners grumble about the meagerness of the portions. But the *nouvelle cuisine vegeterienne* style of cookery that is taught here dictates that portions be small. And the very fact that customers cry for more shows that the food is exceptionally tasty.

With the exception of only one item on the menu, we relished the food unreservedly. This was the Crispy Scallion Pancakes that were so crispy they tasted like hockey pucks. But the entree--Savory Baked Tofu Arame Stir-Fry with a Melange of Mushrooms and Fresh Vegetables in a Sweet and Spicy Sauce Served on a Bed of Lettuce and Crispy Rice Noodles--was divine. And the dessert! The dessert! Five Spiced Roasted Peach Pie with vegan Basil Ice-Cream and Sour Cherry Sauce, was sublime.

While everyone was clamoring for seconds and thirds on the vegan Basil Ice-Cream, the door to the kitchen suddenly swung open, and we saw something that we were not supposed to see. We spied the dessert chef downing a soup bowl filled with gobs of vegan Basil Ice-Cream. That's how good it was!

SUKHADIA'S [v] $$

Counter service	17 West 45th Street
Pan Indian	bet.5th/ 6th Avenues
All Cards	212-395-2552
No alcohol	M-Sa 9am-9pm
www.sukhadia.com	

As the brain drain from India has tilted towards New York, many Indian vegetarian restaurants have sprung up to cater to the tastes of Indian professionals--a preponderance of whom are lacto-vegetarians. "Lacto," unfortunately. is the operative word here. In the evening, most of the dishes are awash with milk, yogurt and cheese; which makes it difficult for the fastidious vegan. We asked the proprietor, Phil Sukhadia, if the chef could make vegan versions of the dishes containing cheese, ghee or yogurt. He said that he would gladly do so. But we had to wait half an hour for him to tell us that there were only two vegan dishes available--Chana Masala and Suki Bhaji. While these dishes were quite tasty, they were not the vegan versions of the Indian entrees that we had requested.

At lunchtime, there is a buffet, which appears to have more non-dairy dishes to choose from, but even some of these may be cooked with yogurt or ghee; so it pays to inquire of the chef or the sous-chef. Phil told us that there were so many Jain customers, who ply their trade in the nearby diamond center, that he had a special menu designed just for them. And, indeed, the Jain menu, which is a sidebar to the main menu, features a number of dishes that are specially prepared for their stringent dietary requirements. For instance, Jains do not eat root vegetables lest they kill the plant or disturb the microbial and insect life that dwell in the root system. Also, their religious dictates prohibit them from eating vegetable-fruits that contain a superabundance of seeds, such as eggplant, lest they ingest the seeds of life. However, poring over the Jain menu and seeing the number of dishes that contained cheese and milk, made us wonder if the vaunted Jain compassion for insects and microbes did not extend to the cow, which is milked remorselessly and whose unwanted male calf is callously turned into veal.

However, what struck us as most odd is that the restaurant should go to great lengths to please Jains, but not do anything to please vegans. Sukhadia's is one of the few Indian lacto-vegetarian restaurants in Manhattan that does not make some concessions to vegans. Madras Cafe for instance, marks vegan dishes with a "V" and has dishes that use soy foods, as does Desi Junction. New York Dosas, is the only Indian restaurant (actually a restaurant on wheels) that is 100% vegan. The desserts at Sukhadia's are almost all tainted with milk, cheese and ghee. Finally, the bill was twice what it should have been. So it definitely repays one's effort to examine one's bill, as well as the bill-of-fare, very, very carefully when dining here.

SULLIVAN STREET BAKERY (PIZZERIA) [v] $

Counter service
Pizzas/baked goods
All cards
No alcohol

533 West 47th Street
bet 10th/ 11th Avenues
212-265-5580
daily 7am-7pm

For lacto-vegetarians who want to go vegan, often the hardest food to give up is Pizza made with cheese. Now at last there is a place that serves vegan pizzas that are every bit as tasty as their non-vegan counterparts. One of them in particular, the Pizza Patate, is so good that Martha Stewart features a recipe for it on her web site. The owner of this bakery-cum-pizzeria, Jim Lahey, actually demonstrated how to make it on Martha's TV show. It's a flat pizza topped with a layer of thinly sliced potatoes. That's how pizzas are done at Sullivan Street. Straightforward and delicious with savory toppings like the sliced Crimini mushrooms of the Pizza Funghi. Or the rosemary, olive oil, and salt of the Pizza Bianca. Or, the cherry tomatoes and basil of the Pizza Pugliesi. Or, the tomato topping of the Pizza Pomodoro. Other pizza toppings vary with the seasons. You're allowed to sample each pizza before ordering one--which could be dangerous because you might end up ordering them all.

Located only a few blocks from the theater district, Sullivan Street is a great place to grab a pre-theater light supper or snack before the show. Seating is severely restricted though. There are only two rickety chairs inside the bakery and two outside. So, if you want to sit down to enjoy your meal, take it to the theater coffee bar and devour it there. Also, if you want condiments on your pizza, you'll have to bring your own. Sullivan Street doesn't furnish any of the extra seasonings that conventional pizza parlors do.

Vegans should watch out for the Zucchini Pizza, it's topped with appetizing Zucchini morsels, but below the top layer is a subcutaneous layer of cheese. And the Tortes are all made with butter. It pays to inquire about the ingredients before biting into anything here.

ZENITH [v] $$

Full service
Asian vegetarian
All major cards
Full bar

311 West 48th Street
bet. 8th/9th Avenues
212-262-8080
daily 11:30am-11:00pm

The zenith of Chinese vegetarian cooking, this restaurant may not be--that distinction belongs to Tien Garden and Vegetarian Dim Sum House, but the portions are generous, the food is tasty and any restaurant that has Zen as the first syllable of its name and serves distinguished vegetarian food is a welcome companion to Zen Palate (on which its name plays) in the theater district. Try the Mango Temptation (fresh sweet mango, vegetarian chicken, fresh peppers & onions sauteed lightly with chef's special mango sweet & sour sauce)as a main course and your palate will reach its zenith for the day. Dessert portions are rather small, (We had the Chocolate Truffle Cake.) which should suit the calorie-conscious dieter. Vegans: watch out for dairy and honey in desserts. Also, vegans should be cautioned that Zenith sharea kitchen and dining facilities with a non-veg. restaurant.

ZEN PALATE [ve]$$ 👍

Full service
Asian vegetarian
All major cards
No alcohol

663 Ninth Avenue
at 46th Street
212-582-1669
daily 11:30am-10:45pm

This Zen Palate stands sentinel at the end of New York's restaurant row, providing the only palatable vegetarian option in the theater district. In the cozy, tastefully decorated interior, we love to dine on a pre-theater repast of Scallion Pancakes as an appetizer, followed by a main course of Mediterranean Medley (artichokes, basil, and tomatoes, stir-fried to perfection in a zesty garlic sauce). For dessert, it is our wont to have their scrumptious Chocolate-Raspberry Reincarnation. Now, properly fed, we're ready to watch the "strutters and fretters" on the boards of Broadway.

See other location under Below Canal Street.

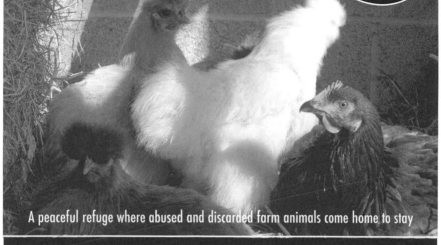
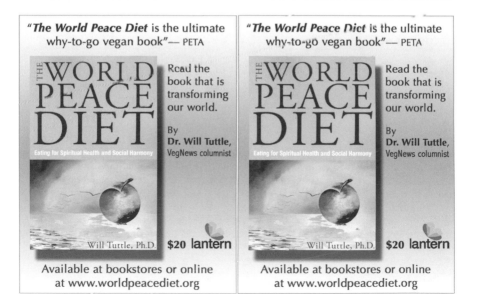

MIDTOWN EAST and Gramercy Park
(East 14th to East 59th Streets)

BODY AND SOUL [ve] **$**

Food stand
International, organic
No cards
No alcohol

Union Square Farmer's Market
at East 17th Street
212-982-5870
M, F 8am-6pm

One of the best ways to keep body and soul together in the city is to have a light vegan meal at the vegan food stand in the Union Square market, which is called aptly enough Body and Soul. Started by the owners of Counter restaurant back in 1994, it draws throngs of hungry folk for breakfast, lunch, early light suppers, and snacks. And it's not hard to see why. The out-size wraps and turnovers are quite toothsome. Try the Saffron Potato wrap which teases the palate with plantain chunks hidden inside. Or try the Spinach Portabello Turnover, which is filled with tofu ricotta, and tastes a bit like a Spinach Lasagna. You might want to complement this with a dairy-free Blueberry Muffin, or a Sweet Potato Muffin. Don't leave the stand without biting into a melt-in-your-mouth Chocolate Brownie, or a Wheat-Free Almond Cookie. Then repair to one of the benches in Union Square Park and have an al fresco meal.

See other location in Brooklyn.

BONOBOS [ve] **$**

Self service
Organic living food, kosher
All cards
No alcohol

18 East 23rd Street
bet. Park Avenue/Broadway
212-505-1200
M-Sa 11:30am-8pm

A vegetarian oasis on the E 23rd Street fast food alley, Bonobos is a unique and delightful deli-style restaurant, serving mostly organic 100% vegan and 100% raw fruits, vegetables, nuts, and seeds. Dine on freshly made, tasty preparations under a huge skylight amid lots of plants. Or order lunch or dinner to go and take it to Madison Park across the street. In any event, the friendly staff will let you sample any prepared food to your heart's content. The prices are very reasonable and there is always a good selection of salads and fresh dressings, nut pates, soups, raw "ice- cream," puddings, and more. Everything is made on the premises with the freshest ingredients. Because Bonobo's food is not cooked it retains the maximum nutritional value and good taste.

Bonobos are awesome healthy pleasure-loving primates who are closest to humans, closer than chimpanzees. Their natural, instinctive diet is primarily fruits vegetables nuts and seeds. Who needs the diet doctors? Bonobs's is kosher and is under strict rabbinical supervision

CHENNAI GARDEN [v] **$$**

Full service
Kosher South Indian / Punjabi
All cards
No alcohol

129 East 27th Street
bet. Park/ Lexington Avenues
212-689-1999
Tu-F 11:30am-10pm
Sa, Su 12pm-10pm

Back in the late 1980s, Pradeep Shinde and Neil Constance, the two owners of this Curry Hill eatery, were among the first to open a kosher Indian vegetarian restaurant in New York. They were so successful that they retired to Orlando to take a flyer in the resort hotel business. They were successful there too, but they found that they pined for the fast tempo of New York City. So much so that they decided to collaborate on another kosher Indian vegetarian restaurant- despite the heated competition.

Their new joint venture is called Chennai Garden. The garden is a more figure of speech (a row of plants that borders the front window), but Chennai is the pre-colonial name of Madras, the cultural capital of South India. And the restaurant breathes the pre-colonial spirit of South India
before the Raj, when flesh food was an anomaly. Our palates were tickled by the Tamarind Pullao (rice perfumed with Tamarind and peanuts), the Bhindi Masala (okra curry) and the Behl Puri (a piquant mix of puffed rice, crisped noodles, onion and cilantro). In a nod to veganism, the Gulab Jamun, a flan which is usually made with powdered milk is made here with a powdered non-dairy mock milk. This makes Chennai garden the only Kosher Indian vegetarian restaurant where one may savor a vegan version of a traditional Indian dessert. The all-you-can-eat lunch buffet for $6.95 is one of New York's best restaurant bargains.

CRISP [v] **$**

Counter service
Middle Eastern
All major cards
No alcohol

684 Third Avenue
at 43rd Street
212-661-0000
daily 10-9

In this mid-Eastern vegetarian restaurant in mid-Eastern Manhattan, the word crisp is actually a euphemism for "falafel." Why substitute the word "crisp" for falafel? we asked the co-owner, Alan Kruvi, "Because falafels, as they are conventionally prepared, are greasy and low-end," says Alan. "Most falafel shops use the same oil. They never change it; they just add more oil to the original batch. We use fresh canola oil, and the oil is changed daily."

And lo it was true: the falafel sandwiches in this sleek falafel,..er "crisp" shack are wonderfully crisp and fresh-tasting. The Basic Crisp arrives packaged in a biodegradable box that is cinched with a pull tab. Pull the tab and the box disgorges an hygienic, delectable falafel sandwich.

There are multiple falafel or "crisp" sandwiches on offer. Unfortunately, the only one that vegans can eat is the Basic Crisp. That's because all the others –the Mexican, the Mediterranean, the Parisian--are suffused in sauces that contain insidious ingredients like butter, milk, and cheese.

On the other hand, the Hummus Bowls, of which there are five, are all impeccably vegan. We had the Hummus Bowl with Sautéed Mushrooms [a concave dish of snowy hummus with a huge dollop of sautéed mushrooms in the center] and was quite fetched by it. Others to choose from include Hummus Bowls with Sautéed Eggplant, with Israeli Salad, and with Roasted Pepper.

Blended teas, sweetened with agave nectar, are paired with each dish. As in all the other falafel shacks in the city, there is the obligatory fresh lemonade served with a sprig of fresh mint.

All the utensils are compostable and bio-degradable. So just by virtue of eating here, one may make an ecological as well as an ethical affirmation, which is gratifying to the conscience as well as to the palate.

FRANCHIA [ve] $$$ 👍

Full Service
Korean -Western fusion
All cards
Oriental & Western Wines and Beers

12 Park Avenue
bet. 34th/ 35th Streets
212-213-1001
daily 11am-10pm

William and Terri Choi, the owners of Hangawi, have opened a tea house on Park avenue and 34th street that rivals Hangawi in elegance. Its name, Franchia, means "free, lavish and generous." Decorated to look like the interior of a Korean country tea house, it provides a refuge from the turmoil and hubbub of the city, where one may sip one's tea in a Zen-like zone of tranquility. Since we happen not to be tea drinkers, it is important to emphasize that one can dine very spaciously here and not drink a drop of tea. But, for those who love tea, Franchia is a tea shrine where one may choose from a wide selection of exotic teas, many of which are purported to have medicinal powers. Try 1st Picked Korean Wild Green Tea from the rocky slopes of Mt. Jilee, or 2nd Picked Mt. Guhwa Green Tea. There is a fixed price Royal Tea Tray, and a Zen Tea Tray. For those who prefer herbal teas, there is Mixed Herbal Tea, a Ginger Tea, a Date Paste Tea, or a Korean Plum Tea.

We chose to consume our tea as a food rather than as a beverage, so we started with Green Tea Pancakes, which were quite yummy. For a main course, we had the Sautéed Soy and Grain Meat With Asparagus and a side order of Green Tea Noodles. Also very yummy. For dessert, we had their incomparable Soy Cheese Cake with a dollop of Raspberry Sorbet.

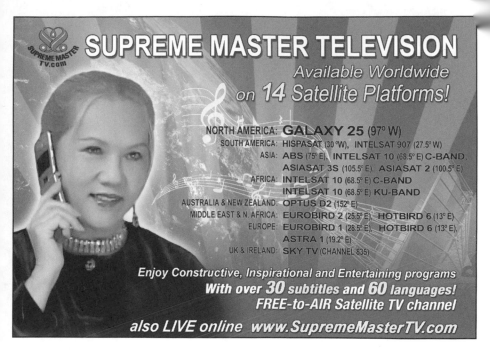
HANGAWI [ve] **$$$**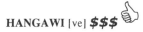

Full service
Korean
All major cards
Oriental and Western wines and beer
Soju cocktails

12 East 32nd Street
bet. Fifth/ Madison Avenues
212-213-0077 ; 212-213-6068
M-F 12pm-3pm, 5pm-10:30pm
Sa 11am-10:30pm, Su 12pm to 10pm

Unless you've spent time in a Korean Buddhist monastery run by Alice Waters, you've never had food like this before. Slip off your shoes, enter a zone of absolute harmony with the sounds of rushing wind and water filling the air, and prepare to be confounded by the menu: grilled lanceolata? Ginseng in a stone bowl? Pumpkin porridge? Date paste tea? The best way to cope with this unfamiliar collection of mountain roots and greens is to order the Emperor's Meal bringing you a sample of such variety most Koreans have never tasted it. The service is impeccable and the flavors are a wonderful assortment of surprises. The owners of this superlative restaurant, William and Terri Choi, are devout Buddhists who come by their ethical vegetarian or vegan philosophy naturally. They are noted for their support of vegetarian and animal rights causes as much as for their devotion to the highest standards in food preparation and service.

35

MADRAS MAHAL |v| $$

Full service
Indian vegetarian, kosher
Major cards
Korean beer & wine

104 Lexington Avenue
bet. 27th/28th Streets
212-684-4010
Su 12pm-10pm, F 11:30am-3pm
M-Th 11:30am3pm & 5:30pm-10pm

The menu asks for your patience since the food is freshly prepared. Maybe that includes scything the wheat for chapatis. At any rate, it took 45 minutes to get drinks and an hour for samosas which were hot and flaky, with the rich taste of freshly ground spices. After another half hour we got Kala Chana (black chick pea curry) and Sukhi Bhaji (potato stir fried with hot pepper, dry fruit and nuts). But we were cranky after waiting so long, and the dishes didn't measure up to our expectations, especially at nine dollars apiece.

MAOZ |v| $

Counter service
Israeli falafel shack, kosher
All Cards
No alcohol
www.maozusa.com

638 Union Square East
bet. 16th/ 17th Streets
212-260-1988
daily 11am-12am

Like a green shoot in a bowl of sprouting chick-peas, Maoz joins the other vegetarian falafel shacks in Manhattan--Crisp, Taim, Hummus Place, Moishes, et al, that have sprung up, seemingly overnight.

Oblong and solidly built, Maoz looks like nothing so much as a bunker, which is exactly what Maoz means in Hebrew. The "bunker" looks eminently capable of fending off carnivorous assaults from the malevolent fast food chains that huddle nearby. Maoz's secret weapon, with which, we predict, it will eventually flatten its carnivorous competitors, is the seductive flavor of its food. Another potent weapon is the undeniable fact that vegetarian fast food is healthful: It's the only fast food that isn't fat food. Rather, it's fit food. Eat as many salads and as many falafel sandwiches as you like and you'll still be slender.

All the food is prepared on the premises. The most popular item on the menu, which accounts for 80 percent of the sales is the Maoz salad, which one may assemble from as many as twenty healthful ingredients. Such as pickled eggplant, pickled carrot salad, couscous with parsley, shredded cabbage, onion and tomato salad, olives and, assorted pickles, special broccoli and cauliflower salads.

Add five falafel balls to the above ingredients, and you can construct a falafel salad. Add five falafel balls, and make yourself a Maoz falafel sandwich. We savored the Maoz Royal, which contained assorted salad ingredients plus eggplant and humus.

Bunkers and vegetarianism would seem to be incompatible notions, but, according to Nat Hirshman and his daughter. there are already 32 vegetarian bunkers in Europe. When you stop to consider it: a bunker is a zone of tranquility, an oasis of peace in a hostile world. And that's what Maoz is--a gustatory peace bunker that promises to spread and swallow New York.

See other locations under East Village and Upper West Side.

PONGAL[v] $$

Full service
Indian vegetarian
Major cards
No alcohol

110 Lexington Avenue
bet. 27th and 28th St.
212-696-9458
M-Th 11:30am-10pm
F-Su 11:30am-10:30pm

Yes, the Big Apple boasts some of the finest Indian vegetarian cuisine this side of the Indus River. Night after night, one can eat in one great Indian restaurant after another without feeling that one has dined redundantly. The dining experience at Pongal is incomparable. Start with appetizers called Kachoori, then progress to a roll-your-own-crepe called Paper Dosa. This is a large Indian crepe made of rice flour and served with spiced potato on the side. The trick to rolling your own crepe is to tear off bits of dosa; fill them with the spicy potato mixture then dip them into a fresh coconut chutney. All dishes are served on banana leaves. Undhiya a Gujarati dish that we sampled is highly recommended containing as it does such exotic ingredients as yam, lotus root potatoes and eggplant. When we'd polished off this and the okra-tomato curry, the waiter brought us Kachooris (deep-fried puffs of Toor dal lentil and Bathata Dada). We finished the meal with a decaf coffee from Madras. We forbore to have any of the tempting desserts as none (alas! alack!) was vegan.

See other location under Upper East Side.

PURE FOOD AND WINE (ve) $$$ 👍

Full service
Gourmet raw food
All cards
Organic beer & wines

54 Irving Place
bet. 17th/ 18th Streets
212-477-1010
M-Su 12pm-3pm
M-Su 5:30pm-11pm

With the opening of Pure Food and Wine the preparation of rawfood has reached its apogee in New York, if not the world. The food, which is 100% vegan and raw, shows off the virtuosity of two talented New York chefs--Sarma Melngailis and Matthew Kenney (formerly of Matthews on the Upper East Side). In previous incarnations, both had won fame as chefs de cuisine cooking animal flesh for carnivores. But suddenly, about two years ago, over dinner at the rawfoods restaurant Quintessence, they had a simultaneous epiphany; they realized that eating vegan rawfood was better for their health, better for the health of animals, and better for the ecological health of the planet. Hence their motto, which they proudly display on the front page of their menu: "Handcrafted flavors that rejuvenate the body, mind, and planet."

A hard-bitten skeptic might scoff that chefs who excelled at making dead animal parts taste yummy should have no trouble infusing raw vegetable and fruit concoctions with flavor. Just so. This is why the food at Pure Food and Wine surpasses that of any other rawfood restaurant that we have visited. These two chefs have applied the hautest techniques of nouvelle cuisine to the preparation of rawfoods, and the results are truly sensational.

We can unreservedly recommend all the dishes that we tasted. Start with the Thai Lettuce Wraps that come with a spicy tamarind dipping sauce. Another appetizer to try is the Tomato Tartare with Kaffir Lime. For a main course, try the Beet Ravioli-- [Rectangles of thinly sliced beets sandwiched together with a cashew nut filling]. Or the Golden Squash Pasta with Summer Black Truffles [Spiralized Yellow Squash slathered with a hearty truffle sauce with sweet peas and chervil]. For dessert, we commend to your tastebuds Chewy Dark Chocolate Cookie with Chocolate and Pistachio Ice Creams [This is a soft cookie, served with candied pistachios, strawberry sauce, and dollops of vegan ice-cream made from nut cream.]

The restaurant's interior is plush, and the walls are decorated with pictures of happy animals (pleased, no doubt, because they're not being eaten). The spacious patio is the perfect setting for the eating of things raw. Here one may dine al fresco, and in the event of a sudden downpour waiters are adept at setting up huge parasols that protect the diners from precipitation. The atmosphere is so convivial that strangers talk to each other across tables. Sitting next to us were two non-vegetarian women who were prolonging their meal by ordering endless glasses of coconut water and organic wine--because they couldn't tear themselves away from the place. It's that magnetic!

Not content to rest on their laurels, Kenney and Melngailis have collaborated on an uncook book, Raw Food/ Real World: 100 Recipes to Get the Glow, which tells one how to reconstruct the dishes that are on offer in the restaurant. Published by Regan Books, it promises well to be a bestseller. Early in 2006, Sharma and Matthew parted ways. Sharma continues to run Pure Food with her customary élan and Matthew has gone on to start a chain of rawfood cafes called Blue Green, which, unfortunately, came a cropper.

PURE JUICE & TAKE AWAY |ve| $$$

Full Service
Gourmet raw food
$4.00-12.00 (all cards)
No alcohol

125 1/2 East 17th Street
bet. 3rd Avenue/ Irving Place
212-477-7151
daily 11am-11pm

This is the vest-picket version of Pure Food and Wine with many of the menu items at PFW available for take-out. Here, you can get one of Pure Food's tastiest dishes, the Heirloom Tomato Lasagna with Basil Pesto and Pignoli Ricotta. Their Flatbread Pizza with Hummus, Avocado and Mint Pesto makes a delectable take away lunch, as does our favorite Tortilla Wrap with Chili Spiced 'Beans' The juice bar offers some exotic juice combinations such as Hot Pink (Beet Pineapple, Watermelon and Ginger) and smoothies. Try the Mango Shake (Mango, Fresh Coconut Water and a dash of Vanilla). Many of the desserts served at Pure Food are also offered here. We were glad to see the Toco Coco Brownies. And we also liked the Fruit, Granola and Vanilla Cream Parfait.

The desserts, as at Pure Food, are made without honey. Making a commendable effort to be consistently vegan, they use Agave Nectar and Maple Syrup instead of honey.

SARAVANA BHAVANA (v) $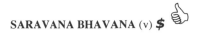

Full service
Chennai homestyle
$6.25-13.95 (major cards)
Wine & beer

81 Lexington Avenue
at 26th Streets
212-679-0204
Lunch Tu-Su 12m-4pm
Dinner 5:30pm-10pm

Saravana Bhavan--Englished means "house of Saravana". Brother of Ganesh, the elephant god of prosperity, Sarvana seems to be shedding a benign protection on this house. And according to the manager, Ms. Ramaya, they will need every ounce of Saravanaas' help. There is fierce competition with other Indian restaurants on Curry Hill, and there appears to be a jinx on the street corner where Saravanaas is located.. So far, every restaurant that has occupied this corner has failed.

But if the quality of the food and the service are anything to go by, Saravanaas will beat the odds. Already, the place is packed with frugal diners, both Indian and Western, who obviously recognize a bargain when they eat one. Modestly priced, and highly flavorsome, the cuisine--Chennai homestyle--is the type of food that one might encounter at a home in Chennai (formerly Madras). The menu abounds in delicious dosas, uthapams, vadas, and thalis redolent of India's deep south. Nearly all the dishes are cooked in oil, not ghee (clarified butter). But vegans must beware of the Iddly (Steamed Rice and Lentil Patty), which is topped off with a ladleful of ghee. Also, the Sambars in the Thalis are sometimes flavored with ghee.

For an appetizer, we had the Sambar Vada (Crispy Lentil Doughnuts in a Mild, Spicy South Indian Soup, Garnished with Onion and Cilantro). For the main course, we had the Dried Fruit Rava Dosa (a mildly spiced Crepe made of Wheat and Rice Flour, blended with Whole Raisins, Pistachios, and Cashews). This we dipped into three different coconut-based chutneys and a sambar. Verboten to vegans are the desserts. As in most Indian restaurants, they are highly caseous, containing ghee, milk, yogurt, and cheese.

Unlike other restaurants on Curry Hill, Saravanaas refuses to use frozen vegetables and will not serve leftovers. Ms. Ramaya told us that all the vegetables are purchased from local Indian suppliers. This accounts for the high quality and astonishing freshness of each dish. Saravana Bhavan is actually the New York branch franchise of a chain of successful Indian vegetarian restaurants that originate in Chennai. So all the dishes are made to standards set by the home office in Chennai. This can have its drawbacks. When we asked for soy milk to be used in a Lassi, or in an Indian coffee, which is pre-mixed with cow's milk, the manager told us that the home office does not permit its franchises to substitute soy milk for cow's milk. This strikes us as a silly practice-- especially as the home office has allowed the New York franchise to serve wine and beer, which no other restaurant in the chain is allowed to do. So, it is incumbent that vegans politely demand soy milk for their lassis and coffees.[If the Starbucks chain,--which is non-veg.-- can offer soymilk, then why not Saravana Bhavana, which is veg.?] Apart from this notable lapse, the service is faultless, and the food is very good value for the money.

TIFFIN WALLAH |v| $

Counter service	127 East 28th Street
Mumbai homestyle	bet. Park/ Lexington Avnues
All Cards	212-685-7302
Beer & wine	M-Su 11:30am-3:00am
www.tiffinwallah.us	M-Su 5pm-110pm

What is a tiffin wallah.? We asked Pradeep Shinde, owner of this eating establishment of the same name. An institution peculiar to Mumbai--which is where Pradeep grew up.--"tiffin wallah," is a man who fetches vegetarian lunches made by Mumbai housewives; he then ferries them to their husbands in their city offices. Pradeep wanted to import this concept to New York in a slightly modified form. So he sees the restaurant as a sort of communal "tiffin wallah," conveying homestyle vegetarian meals to New York City's office workers.

Trained as an engineer in Mumbai, Pradeep moved to New York where he switched his

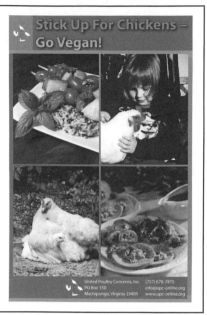

major to hotel management at NYU. For a time, after his graduation, he worked as a personal butler at the Park Lane Hotel. Then, he started his own restaurant, Madras Mahal, which was the first vegetarian restaurant on Curry Hill. (Now there are seven.)

Tiffin Wallah hums with efficiency. Pradeep is everywhere at once, recalling his buttling days; he bustles about, overseeing the minutest detail. He wipes a spot of gravy from a bin cover, then he replenishes the salad bowls. A small but diligent wait staff is poised to do his bidding.

At lunch, the place is thronged with young, and middle-aged professionals who rhapsodize over the six-dollar buffet--the best luncheon deal in town. When we asked him how long he would peg the price at six dollars, Pradheep promised us, perhaps with a touch of hyperbole, that this price would be fixed in perpetuity.

On weekends, Tiffin Wallah serves exotic dosas (crepes) that cannot be found anywhere else. We recommend the Pesaratu, a dosa made from green lentils and green chilies; the Spring Dosa, which is a mixed vegetable dosa; and the Jaipur Masala Dosa.

At the buffet, we could eat only the Chana Masala, and a vegetable sabji. The other dishes, save for the delicious, small stuffed vegetable Uttapam, were caseous. Since many of our readers are persnickety vegans, as we are, they are reluctant even to eat in places where mammary secretions are served. So we extracted from Pradeep a promise that he would be willing to make mock meat substitutions for any caseous a la carte item. We urged him to visit Desi Junction, which, albeit a working-man's Indian restaurant, they nonetheless have integrated soy into a number of their formerly caseous dishes.

VATAN [v] $$$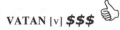

Full service
Indian
$31.00 prix fixe (V, MC)
Full bar

409 Third Avenue
at 29th Street
212-689-5666 (reservations essential)
Tu-Su 5:30pm-10pm
Closed Mondays

At first glance, $31.00 *prix fixe* may seem like a lot of rupees, but think of a visit to Vatan as a cut-price ticket to India. The decor instantly transports you to a village in Gujarat, where costumed waiters and waitresses look as if they've just popped out of Aladdin's lamp to do your bidding. At the snap of your fingers, they will bring you all the appetizers you can eat; and the appetizers are so indescribably scrumptious, you'll eat yourself into a stupor. We stuffed ourselves unashamedly with delicate miniature samosas filled with peas and potatoes, the Chana Masala (chick peas with onions and coriander) and an array of Indian breads such as papadams and puris, but still found room for a rich dessert of Mango Rus (mango pulp). The music, authentic Indian ragas, is soft and unobtrusive. The food is prepared with canola oil, not ghee. The service is faultless.

ZEN BURGER [v] $

Counter service
Healthful fast food
All Cards
No alcohol

465 Lexington Avenue
bet. 45th/ 46th Streets
212-661-6080
M-Sa 10am-9pm

Former Wall Street money manager, James Tu, who used to manage 350 million a year in assets, has been a vegetarian for nine years only, but after he went veg. he decided to invest in a chain of restaurants purveying healthful and tasty veg. fast food. It has taken nearly eight years for him to bring it to birth. We, along with a number of Wall Street specialists were invited to a pre-launch party in which we sampled some of the food that would be on offer at the soon-to-be opened Zen Burger. Even deep-dyed carnivorous types, among the analysts, had to admit that Zen Burger's food had captured the texture as well as the appealing flavor of fast food. The Zen Burger with its side of Yam Fries was also highly successful and is one of the fastest selling items on the Zen Burger menu in 2009. We are also fond of their Shanghai Tofu Wrap (tofu, hoisin sauce, lettuce, cucumber, carrots and onion in a spinach wrap). For dessert, we always have their All Natural Non-Dairy Sundae (vanilla, chocolate, swirl non-dairy soft serve with chocolate topping, sprinkles and nuts). Our favorite beverages are their Izzi water, and their Lemon Ginger Green Tea.

In taking Zen Burger national, Mr.Tu is not aiming specifically for the steadfast vegetarian customer, who represents only 2.3% of the population (up from 1% in 1994), but for the flexitarians (part-time vegetarians) which represent 25% of the US population. We concur with the opinion of the stock analysts who sampled his food, Tu's Zen Burger is a definite boy!

GREENWICH VILLAGE

(Houston Street to West 14th Street, Hudson River to Fifth Avenue)

EAST-WEST CAFE [v] **$**

Self service
Organic Asian-Western cuisine
All cards
Organic beer & wine
www.eastwestnyc.com

78 Fifth Avenue
bet. 13th/ 14thStreets
212--243-3667
daily 10am-9pm

By the time it closed its doors for good in November 2005, the old East West bookstore--an endearingly shabby esoteric book shop--must have laid up masses of good karma in its checkered life. For now, under the new ownership of Jan Matthews, it has attained a much higher incarnation as an elegantly designed metaphysical book shop with a spiffy new cafe upstairs--the East West Cafe.

Chad Currier, the manager of the East West Cafe, said that he tried to make the cafe "a culinary manifestation of the spirit of the bookstore." In this he has succeeded admirably. The space fairly exhales spirituality.

Poised above the bookstore, on the cloud-like mezzanine floor, we ate our meal while we gazed down on the patrons below--as if we were lesser Hindu deities. Speaking of deities--gorgeous pen and ink drawings illustrating mythological scenes from the Mahabharata, the Ramayana, and other Indian epics, grace the cafe's walls. [Copies of these drawings are for sale.]

Suitably enough, many of the main dishes have Sanskrit names as if the very act of consuming them were an act of devotion. We had a delicious Capanata Salad (triple-washed spinach, alfalfa sprouts, vine-ripe tomatoes, grilled eggplant, garbanzos, roasted garlic, oil-cured olives) followed by a Tuscan Roasted Vegetable Sandwich that featured roasted eggplant sun-dried tomato, triple-washed spinach, organic apple, and basil on seven-grain bread. To accompany it, we sipped the most delicious
Soy Chai (black tea, soymilk with agave nectar, and Indian masala).

After eating to repletion, we pursued one of our favorite postprandial pastimes--browsing in a bookstore. Only now we had but to descend the staircase to have a browse in New York's best metaphysical bookstore. Although the cafe upstairs is meant to be subservient to the bookstore--its food is so appealing, and its space so seductively designed, that eventually it may upstage the bookstore to become a destination for vegan gourmets.

GOBO [ve]$$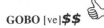

Full service
Organic, Asian-Western fusion cuisine
All cards
Organic beer & wine
www.goborestaurant.com

402 Sixth Avenue
at 8th Street
212-255-3242
Su-We 11:30am-11:30pm
Th-Sa 11:30am-12am

The atmosphere of Gobo-- the Japanese word for the root vegetable, burdock--is reminiscent of the tastefully decorated Zen Palate restaurants. The comparison is entirely appropriate because the owners of Gobo, Darryn and David Wu are the sons of the owners of Zen Palate, Mr. and Mrs. Tiehjyh Wu. Just as Zen Palate invokes the influence of Buddhism as their raison d' etre, so there is a statue of the Buddha prominently displayed at Gobo; he is smiling his blessing upon Gobo food, which is faithful to the Buddha's first precept of ahimsa (non-violence to all living creatures).

Gobo is proof of the fact that one can be a principled vegetarian yet enjoy the most exquisite food. For the food at Gobo's outstrips the cuisine of its parent restaurant Zen Palate. (This is ironic because most of the dishes were created by Mrs. Wu, the co-owner of Zen Palate). We started our dinner with a smoothie called The Awakening (mango, cherry and wolfberry), which was truly ambrosial. With our taste buds duly awakened, we were in a fit condition to enjoy the entrees, which were also very much to our taste--Sizzling Soy Cutlet Platter with Black Pepper Sauce, and the Soy Filet with Coconut Curry Rice. The desserts, all of which are vegan, were also extraordinary. We relished the Multi-layered Chocolate Cake and the Coconut-Chocolate Pudding with Mango Puree.

There are two non-vegan dishes--Avocado Tartare, which contains honey; and Crispy Spinach and Soy Cheese Wontons, which contains casein, a cows' milk extract, and egg, an ingredient in the won ton wrappers. Cow's milk, alas, is also available to tea and coffee drinkers who prefer it to the soy milk that is on offer.

The talk is that, if it is successful, Gobo plans to franchise the restaurant. Judging from the impeccable service, the attractive decor and the exquisite food, the burdock will soon be taking root in other American cities.

See other location in Upper East Side.

HUMMUS PLACE [v]$

Full Service
Israeli vegetarian, kosher
All cards
Wine & Beer

99 Macdougal Street
bet. W. 3rd/ Bleecker Streets
212-533-3089
Su-Th 11am-12am
Fr-Sa 11am-2am

New York already has single-food-item restaurants dedicated to the French Fry, the Falafel, the Baked Potato, the Crepe, the Dosa, the Pancake, the Doughnut, Popcorn, Soup, and the

Noodle; there is even a Candy bar (Dylan's)--so why not a restaurant devoted soley to Hummus? At Hummus Place, a tidy little beanery with walls the color of tahini, you can order two different styles of hummus--one made from fava beans and chickpeas, Hummus Foul (pronounced fool), and the other made from whole chickpeas, Hummus Masabacha. The fava beans and the chickpeas are imported from Israel to insure quality and freshness. The beans are then set to soak overnight and are chopped up in a huge Robotcoupe; then cooked for a full five hours. The hummus is served with a snow white tahini which is also imported from Israel.Two of the dishes are made with eggs; so vegans must tell the chef to hold the eggs!

Fittingly enough, the man who founded Hummus Place is an Israeli named Ori Apple, formerly of Kibbutz Maoz Haim. After his army service in Israel, Apple alighted in the Big Apple to study cooking at the French Culinary Institute in Soho. Having worked for a number of restaurants and a catering service in the city, Apple decided to strike out on his own. With the help and advice of his best friend--(now co-owner and chef of Hummus Place)--Nitzan Raz, Apple started Hummus Place. Apple's hummus is considered to be so authentic that Israelis joke that they no longer have any reason to visit Tel Aviv.

Because they've been cooked to a fare-thee-well-well, the flavor of the hummuses are a bit bland. Luckily, they come with a hot sauce on the side with a secret recipe whose base is cilantro. We found that the judicious seasoning of hummus with hot sauce enlivens the flavor and makes it go down much better. The hummus also comes with an Israeli Salad (whose ingredients are not imported from Israel). To give it an added fillip, we tried mixing the Israeli Salad in with the hummus and the hot sauce Then we used; the resultant mixture to fill a whole wheat pita pocket, which came with our order. This worked splendidly. We washed it all down with a cool glass of refreshing lemonade (also made with a secret recipe) that contains a sprig of fresh Israeli Mint. At the end of our meal, we left feeling satisfied and full of beans.

See other locations under East Village and Upper West Side.

INTEGRAL YOGA NATURAL FOODS [ve] $

Take out counter
International
All cards
No alcohol
www. iynaturalfoods.com

229 West 13th Street
bet. 7th/ 8th Avenues
212-243-2642
M-F 9am-9:30pm
Sa-Su 9-8:30pm

Integral Yoga was started by Swami Satchidananda back in the seventies. The Swami taught that it was bad karma to consume or purvey animal flesh. Consequently, Integral Yoga is one of the few health food stores in the city that doesn't peddle flesh. Now you can tap into their good karma by having a meal there. Nestled into the North West corner of the store is one of the city's best vegan buffets. You may choose from such selections as Curried Black-Eyed Peas, Hot and Spicy Tofu and Bokchoy with Almonds. There is also a juice bar where you may purchase soups and veggie burgers. If you're a rawfoodist, take heart! There's a capacious salad bar, and in a refrigerated display case next to the buffet, there is an appetizing selection of raw vegetable pies, fruit pies, cakes, and cookies.

JIVAMUKTEA CAFE [ve] *$$* 👍

Counter Service
Global vegan organic
All cards
No alcohol

841 Broadway (2nd Fl.)
bet. 13th/ 14th Streets
212-353-0214
M-F 11am-9pm
Sa-Su 1am-6pm

Overlooking the hubbub of Broadway in a spacious, airy setting, with an azure ceiling, antique chandeliers. and soaring stained glass windows, the new JivamukTea Café is housed inside the Jivamukti Yoga Center, which, from an ethical standpoint, is the best school of yoga in the city.

Unlike most yoga ashrams that give short shrift to *ahimsa,* which is the first precept of all classical yoga systems. it is clear that Jivamukti's founders, Sharon Gannon and David Life, uphold the view of Patanjali that if one is to advance spiritually in yoga one must eat non-violent food. In fact, in a recent interview, Sharon Gannon said," Veganism is essential to the practice of yoga, where you do not exploit animals for any purpose. Patanjali in the *Yoga Sutras,* gives *ahimsa* (non-harming of others) as the primary means to enlightenment." To that end, Sharon Gannon has created a menu that is conducive to attaining the higher states of yogic consciousness—and to having a transcendent dining experience.

This JivamukTea Café is figuratively a reincarnation of the first JivamukTea Cafe, which was managed by star chef Matthew Kenney, and went defunct not long after it opened. However, this new incarnation promises to have more staying power because it is that much better than its predecessor, which tried too hard to be trendy. This one's recipes come from co-founder Sharon Gannon's home kitchen, so they have a familial, home-style air to them.

We tried their most popular sandwich, the Grilled Portobello Panino (portabella mushroom, sweet onions, nutritional yeast, chimchurri sauce on grilled sourdough). Yummy! Then we proceeded to have the Montana Salad, which contains seasonal vegetables, lettuce, cucumbers, black beans, quinoa, sprouts grown on the premises--all of it suffused with a turmeric-tahini dressing. Heavenly! To wash it down, we chugged a 3rd Eye Smoothie (acai, coconut water, banana, and organic vanilla extract). Ambrosial! For dessert, we had the Walnut Cake and the oversized Chocolate Chip Cookie that had just been plucked from the oven--with the result that the chips were still gooey and the dough was still soft and friable. Celestial! It was a vegan Toll House Cookie raised to a higher order of cookie. After dessert, as we watched the sunlight shimmering through the stained glass, we sipped, meditatively two generous cups of Love Blend Tea, a black tea with subtle chocolate overtones.

In spite of all the delicious food we had eaten, we seemed to float on air as we left the café, mumbling a *sotto voce* M-m-m-m-m mingled with Om-m-m-m-m-m.

👍 Indicates we especially recommend this restaurant for the quality of the food.

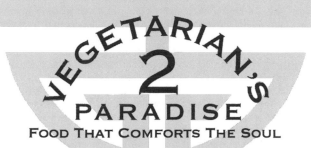
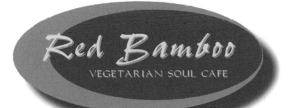

NEW YORK DOSAS|ve|$ 👍

Food cart
South Indian
No cards
No alcohol

Washington Square Park
West 4th/ Sullivan Streets
917-710-2092
M-Sa 11am-5pm

We had to stand in line behind ten people to give our order to Thiru Kumar, the chef who works his magic at this outdoor food cart. Our order was for a Masala Dosa (a rolled rice-flour crepe stuffed with spicy potato mixture), Jafna Dosa (a rolled rice-flour crepe stuffed with Sambahl); Ponidicherry Utapam (a flat bread topped with fresh, chopped vegetables); and Iddly with Sambar (an Indian biscuit made from lentil flour and dipped in a spicy Sambar or soup).

Thiru, a native of Sri Lanka, works fast; he pours a batter made from crushed fermented rice and lentils on the griddle and within a few seconds, Utapam and Dosas appear, as if by magic. He fills them with spicy mashed potatoes and chopped fresh vegetables--and the result dosas and utapams worthy of the finest Indian restaurants.

Thiru packed our order into boxes; then we sat on a bench in Washington Square park and savored every morsel.

It's hard to believe that so much food can pour forth from one little food cart! In addition to the Dosas, one may order Samosas with vegetable fillings; Medhu Vada (lentil donuts), and the aforementioned Iddly with Sambar. Thiru also offers up a unique array of tinned fruit juices imported from Thailand--such as Rambutan juice, Longan juice, and, our favorite, Lychee juice--that are available nowhere else in the city. Unusual for an Indian food establishment, vegans may dine here without having to ask about objectionable ingredients--as all the food is 100 per cent vegan. [Thiru bowed to pressure from vegan students at the NYU Vegan Society to make his food cart exclusively vegan. Now he himself has turned vegan.]

RED BAMBOO |ve| $$ 👍

Full service
Asian soul food fusion
All cards
No alcohol
www.redbamboo-nyc.com

140 West 4th Street
bet. 6th/MacDougal
212-260-1212
M-F 4pm-12am
Sa-Su 12pm-12am

"Soul Food with Asian overtones" is how the proprietor, Jason Wong, the son, of the owners of VP2, describes the cuisine At play here are multi-ethnic flavors such as Chinese, Korean, Thai, Indian. Creole and Soul Food. In most instances, the fusion of flavors works.

For appetizers, we had the Jerk Spiced Seitan, which was tangy and tasty, as were the Deep-Fried Butterfly Shrimp, and the gluten "pork" in the Tonkatsu Chops. We also sampled the Tandoori Chicken Supreme. and Buffalo Wings, which were finger lickin' good. However, on the debit side, the Seoul Pancake was too mushy and the sweet corn mashed potatoes were way too bland. We capped it all off with a scrumptious Chocolate Peanut Butter Cake served with a dollop of vegan Mint Chocolate Chip ice-cream. The waiters were attentive and hovering.

The only difficulty that vegans might have with eating at Red Bamboo is that the menu is so unrelievedly mock-carnivorous that the mere sight of dishes with names like Tandoori Chicken, Shrimp, and Salmon, no matter how mock, might conjure unpleasant associations with the real thing. Nonethless, Red Bamboo is a great place to take your meat-eating friends to show them how animal flesh may be mocked to perfection. Two dishes contain dairy and these are noted on the menu.

See other location in Brooklyn

SACRED CHOW [v]$$ 👍

	227 Sullivan Street
Full service	bet. West 3rd & Bleecker Streets
International & bakery	212-337-0863
V, AE, MC	M-F 9 am--11pm
Organic beer & wine	Sa-Su 11:30am-11pm
www.sacredchow.com	

Cliff Preefer, the owner of Sacred Chow used to be the head chef as well as the pastry chef, at Candle Cafe back in the mid-90's. Then he decided to strike out on his own and start a veg. delicatessen, which eventually gave place to this new restaurant of the same name. Casting about for a name for his eatery, he hit upon the inspired pun--"sacred chow." With its logo of the meditating cow, and its pun on sacred cow, could Cliff's restaurant have been anything but vegan? Unfortunately, yes. Cliff does serve dairy products in the shape of ice-cream and creamers for coffee. This is rather a desecration of that poor sacred cow, who is exploited for its exudate, is it not?

Apart from this notable lapse, there is an admirable respect for the cow that pervades the restaurant and its menu. There are usually about thirty vegan tapas on offer. The ones we sampled were extraordinary--Korean Tofu Cutlets, the Shredded Tofu Spa Salad, and Curried Steamed Broccoli. The Hero Sandwich that we had as a main course --Roasted Black Olive Seitan, with molten vegan Mozzarella --was so good that we had to stifle a shout of jubilation. [Fact is: Cliff's Hero sandwiches and pastries are so sought-after that he retails them to other snackeries around the city--like the one in the cafe at the Angelika Cinema.]

While we munched our Heroes, amid the warm, rouge tints of the interior decor, we sipped one of Cliff's frozen smoothies, which he calls Gym Body (bananas, toasted almonds, cinnamon, flax oil and apple juice). This was so satisfyig that we could easily have made a meal of it.

For dessert we inhaled Cliff's famous Velvet Triple Chocolate Brownie with a side scoop of organic vegan Raspberry Ice-Cream. Cliff, [excuse the bad pun], we will be dropping over quite often, (especially if S. C. becomes 100% vegan).
• On a recent visit, [2009] we were delighted to learn that Sacred Chow has gone completely

vegan! Did our caustic review have anything to do with their eliminating the mammary secretions from their meun? We fervently hope so! Kudos to Cliff.

'sNICE [v] $

	45 8th Avenue
Self service	at 4th Street
Sandwiches, salads, baked goods	212-645-0310
All cards	daily 7:30am-10pm
Beer & wine	

'sWonderful, 'sMarvelous, 'sNice? You'll surely agree that this coffee shop-cum-bistro deserves a loftier superlative than merely nice. Really, the food is nothing short of 'sMarvelous! That was our original evaluation of 'sNice during the first three years of its existence. Now, we're chagrined to report that, we've detected a dropoff in quality, which seems to have coincided with 'sNice's expansion into Park Slope, Brooklyn. Gone are the board games, children's toys, the Fizzi waters, and the vivid-tasting wraps that we used to adore. We've taken a number of our friends there over the past year. To a person, they've complained that the smoothies, the wraps and the clumps of salad served with them are insipid-tasting and monotonous. "The wraps smack of a doughy blandness with a sameness of flavor," said they. We are reluctantly forced to concur. Perhaps most off-putting of all, though, is the owner's attitude towards veganism, which is one of thinly disguised hostility. When asked if he would ever remove the honey, milk, Brie Cheese, Cream Cheese, Gorgonzola Cheese, Bleu Cheese, Goat Cheese, Mozzarella Cheese, Swiss Cheese, Parmesan Cheese, [Hey! Eight varieties of cheese on the menu! Is this a veg. bistro or a cheese shop?] and other mammary secretions from his menu, he bristled with indignation, and said "Never!"

'sOkay, 'sBland, 'sCheesy, but not 'sMarvelous, as it used to be. Let's hope that he may return to his former high standards, and go vegan!

TAIM [v] $

Counter service	222 Waverly Place
Kosher Israeli falafel shack	at 7th Avenue
All cards	212-691-1287
No alcohol	M-Su 11am-10:30pm
www.taimnyc.com	

According to our researches, the first bona fide vegetarian Israeli falafel shack in NYC is this diminutive Greenwich Village spot caled Taim. Since it was opened by Einat Admony, Taim's lady chef, two years ago, a number of others have sprung up, apparently, in imitation. Ashkara on East Houston Street and Moaz on Union Square East. Curiously enough, none of the owners of these ovo-lacto vegetarian falafel shacks is a vegetarian. They purvey vegetarian food simply because it is more expedient, more healthful, and hygienic to do so.

"Taim," which means delicious in Hebrew, is aptly named. "Taim" was practically every dish we tried here. We particularly relished the Falafel Sandwich. A pita pocket was filled with our choice of Green, Red or Harissa falafel balls and presented to us with side dishes of Israeli salad, pickled green cabbage, and tahini. The pickled carrot and beet salads were pleasingly tart

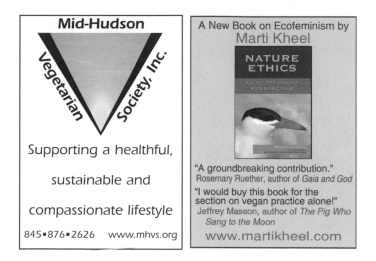
and tasty. We also savored the Sabich (a pita sandwich of fried eggplant, slathered with pickles, onions, tahini and two types of hot sauce. The Sabich was invented by the Lord Sandwich of Israel-- Oved, a one-name-only denizen of the Tel Aviv suburb, Givatayim. It has since become the most popular hand-held food item in Israel. However, before ordering the Sabich, it is important to tell the chef to hold the eggs, because for some strange reason, a chick embryo is felt to be an obligatory ingredient in this dish.

We really liked their home-made French fries that we would rank second only to those of Freedom Tripodi of FoodSwings in Williamsburg. We tossed off a delicious Strawberry-Raspberry-Thai-Basil smoothie, and a Ginger-Mint lemonade, which could make this place one of the city's better juice bars, were it not drenched in milk. However, they use whole and skim milk in their smoothies, so vegans should ask that the blender be washed, before making a non-dairy smoothie, to expel any caseous residues/ The service staff will honor your request with alacrity.

VP2 |v| **$$**

Full service
Chinese
AE,MC,V
No alcohol

140 / 144 West 4th Street
bet. Sixth Ave/ MacDougal Street
212-260-7130/7141
MTh 12pm11pm, F-Sa 12pm-12am

We know, you've long since given up ordering Peking Spare Ribs, Sweet and Pungent Pork and Squid in Black Bean Sauce. Do it anyway. The meaty names just help identify traditional Chinese dishes that VP's Buddhist chefs prepare exclusively without animal products (using soy, wheat, and arrowroot substitutes). The food is authentic and reasonably priced, served in a modern, sleek restaurant . One of the best of this type of place.

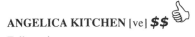

ANGELICA KITCHEN |ve| **$$** 300 E 12th Street

Full service   at Second Avenue
Natural   212-228-2909
No cards   daily 11:30am-10:30pm
No alcohol

Hands down one of the best vegan restaurants anywhere. For 25 years Angelica Kitchen has set the standard for fresh organic fare with a conscience.

Each day there are two very special, always new, special entrees such as "Here Today-- Gone Tamale'" (Festive tamales made with Iroquois white corn masa and roasted home-made seitan, chipotle and ancho chili peppers, all wrapped in a corn husk served with tomato-cilantro salsa, over a baby lima bean sauce, with baby lettuces and steamed local asparagus). Or try the norimake rolls with grilled tempeh, home-made pickled carrots and brown rice; like sushi, they're rolled in nori seaweed .

For those who wish to try Angelica Kitchen's tasty dishes at home, the Angelica Home Kitchen Cookbook by Leslie McEachern (the owner) is for sale in the restaurant. It includes over 100 recipes from the menu archives that have been specially formulated for the home cook. The book also sets forth Leslie's philosophy and principles for running a socially conscious business, and it features profiles of the farmers and artisans who provide the restaurant with the ingredients for their delicious fare.

Angelica's is a dessertatarian's delight. We swooned over the rhubarb layer cake with strawberry frosting and the coconut flan with pineapple salsa was unforgettable. Consistently fresh, flavorful and satisfying, the whole vital menu proves why the outstanding reputation of Angelica Kitchen is so richly deserved Take-out next door.

CAFE VIVA [A.K.A. VIVA HERBAL PIZZERIA] [v] $

Counter service
Italian, organic, kosher
All cards
No alcohol

179 Second Avenue
bet. 11th / 12th Streets
212-420-8801
daily 11am-11pm
Sa-Su 11am-12am

See description under Upper West Side

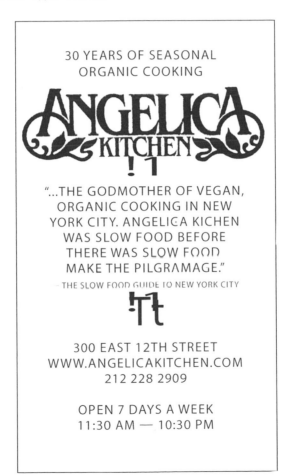

CARAVAN OF DREAMS [ve] *$$* 👍

Full service
International organic, kosher
V,MC
Full bar, organic beer & wine

405 East 6th Street
bet. First Ave/Avenue A
212-254-1613
MSu 11am11pm, Sa 11am-12am
Sa,Su brunch 11am-5pm

Organic vegetarian food in a hippy atmosphere of long hair, mix and match furniture and live music almost every night. Quite relaxing during non-peak hours. No dairy is used; a few years ago, Caravan went completely vegan. Black bean chili, grilled polenta, African spinach stew over rice, pasta, burritos, quesadilla, ginger curried stir fry, tempeh, large salads, sandwiches, "greens of the day." A pleasure. Recently Caravan has begun serving raw-food entrees every day. It also serves a range of raw soups and desserts. Their raw broccoli soup is simply delicious, and their raw raspberry cake bears comparison with any baked cake in town. Every night, their new raw chef creates live food specials that rotate every week. We enjoyed the Taco Salad, the Live Mock Meat Balls, the Live Nachos, and the Live Sandwich. Obviously Caravan's Dreams have come to life.

COUNTER [v] *$$$*

105 First Avenue
bet. 6th Avenue/7th Street
212-982-5870
M-F 5pm-11:30pm
Sa 11am-12am, Su 11am-11pm

Full Service
International, organic
All cards
Organic wines

Counter is a felicitous name for a vegetarian restaurant because it runs counter to the majority of restaurants in New York where dead animals are the focus of dining rituals.

Counter doesn't look counter-cultural though. The handsome interior design with its art deco accents, make it one of New York's most elegant eateries. And the food is sublime. We started with a Porccini Pizza, topped with a nut cheese which was robust and flavorful. We followed this with a Cauliflower Risotto, which were also very tasty. Then we split a Cosmo Burger, a walnut-tempeh patty that was more mundane than cosmic. The garlic-herb aoili that accompanied it was good, but the French-Fries were limp and soggy. For the main course, we recommend the Pasta with Pine Nuts, seasoned with Micro Pepper Cress, picked from Deborah, the owner's roof garden. We were lucky to have dined there on Tuesday, which was raw food night. The raw food chef, Michelle Thorne, prepared a Marinated Peach Salad that was tasty, tart, and sweet. It too was seasoned with herbs from Deborah's roof garden. The raw entree was Stuffed Zucchini Blossoms, which was as flavorful as it was inventive.. The desserts were just as successful. The Verona Chocolate Pie with Vanilla Soy Ice-Cream was eminently satisfying . and we adored their Three Berry Cake,which is topped with a rich vanilla nut cream to compound the decadence. Sad to report, when we quizzed the owners as to whether Counter was totally vegan, they said that it was. Evidently they had forgotten about the milk that they use in the cappuccino, coffees, teas, and other beverages. Deborah assured us that this was an oversight, but that they never used dairy products in any of their food preparations Nonetheless, when it comes to ordering coffee, or Tecchino, a vegan cappuccino, vegans should request soy milk substitutions.

• As of this writing, 2009, a recent visit to Counter disclosed, to our horror, they are not even pretending to be vegan. Cheese, egg, and dairy dishes are conspicuously featured on the menu, as if in defiance of vegan sensibilities, so we've had to strip them of their ranking.

CURLY'S VEGETARIAN LUNCH |v| $$

328 East 14th Street
Full Service   bet. 1st & 2nd Avenues
American fast food   212-598-9998
All cards   Daily 11am-11pm
Beer & Sangria

Rectangular in shape, with cream-colored walls, decorated with two parallel mango stripes, and a lozenge-shaped mirror, there is nothing kinky about Curly's Vegetarian Lunch--except the curly French fries-and the Cubano Sandwich. They have a kinky flavor that wraps itself around your tongue and won't let go. As a rule, we don't care much for mock meat--it's too rereminiscent of the real thing--but we're making an exception for Curly's Cubano. Heaven help the folks who eat the real (carnivorous) Cubano: it has enough cholesterol to thrombose a regiment of Visigoths. But Curly's vegan Cubano with its mock ham, mock dark meat, mock cheese, sans casein, and pickle has a raffish appeal to the taste buds that is not to be denied. Ditto for the mock Buffalo wings. Both by the way are "two-hanky" specials that require two or more napkins to eat without spotting one's blouse. We also savored the Cashew Sofrito (Unsalted cashew nuts in a sofrito of tomato, peppers, olives and achiote. served over fried plantain with back beans and grain). And you don't have to go anywhere else for dessert. Curly's serves a full complement of Vegan Treats' pies and cakes that Veg-City Diner was famous for.

Curly's Vegetarian Lunch seems a quirky name for a restaurant. But a glance at the back page of the menu explains everything. There, the founders and owners of Curly's--David and Jean--have thoughtfully provided the story of how the restaurant got its name. Curly, the grandfather of David, owned a diner in New Hampshire. After a catastrophic flood washed away most of the town, Curly provided free food for the townspeople, and became a local hero. David, wanted to pay tribute to his grandfather's food as well as his unsung heroism.

We almost forgot to mention that Curly's is the brainchild of David and his wife Jean, the former owners of the late-lamented Veg-City Diner, which was forced to close because of a freak kitchen fire. Neither David nor his wife is a vegetarian, but they love to prepare vegetarian food, and delight in inventing new ways to use mock meats. David is also the former owner of Burritoville, the only Mexican restaurant in New York City that has vegan sour cream; he has an abiding love affair with Mexican cuisine. His contract with the buyers of Buttitoville won't let him make Mexican food at Curly's. His vegan Cubano is an homage to the Vegan Mexican cuisine of his heart's desire. Someday, he promises to open a 100 per cent vegan Mexican restaurant. On that day, we'll be the first in line.

HUMMUS PLACE |v| $

Full Service
Israeli vegetarian, kosher
All cards
Wine & Beer

109 St. Marks Place
bet. 1st & A Avenues
212-529-9198
Su-Th 11am-12am
Fr-Sa 11am-2am

See description under Greenwich Village, and other location under Upper West Side.

JUBB'S LONGEVITY |ve| $$

Counter service
Organic Lifefood
V, MC
No alcohol

508 East 12th Street
bet. Avenues A/B
212-353-5000
daily 10am -9pm

Although Jubb's Longevity is technically a deli, so many people crowd into it for lunch, brunch and dinner that we're treating it as a restaurant. The proprietor, Dr. David Jubb, is probably the only chef in New York with a Ph.D in bionutrition. But when it comes to preparing raw food, or "Lifefood," as he calls it, David is an alchemist.

By Lifefood he means food that is organic, unhybridized and uncooked. It's prepared in a way that the "life-force" remains intact, making it easily digestible. Lifefooders eat mainly fruits, nuts and seeds produced by shade-bearing plants that promote the growth of topsoil, thereby enhancing vitality of earth and self. On our last visit to Jubb's, we had the raw pizza, which consists of a sour dough pizza crust made from sprouted buckwheat (actually a seed), flaxseed and low-temperature-dried-sea vegetables, topped with Italian-flavored tomato and pesto sauce with a pine nut and pumpkin seed cheese. We chased this with a glass of cold pressed nut milk and followed that with a vegan live yogurt made from sweetsop and passion fruit for dessert. On our previous visit, we had polished off the Live Burger Deluxe, which is composed of zucchini, celery pine nuts, sprouted pumpkin seeds, sea vegetables, and dehydrated wild fruits and greens. It's served on unleavened sour dough bread on a bed of chopped greens. It comes with a raspberry mayonnaise, a pine nut seed cheese and a spicy sauce. All the ingredients of his dishes, it bears repeating, are organic and raw. For dessert, we downed an antioxidant energy bar made from rose hips, hibiscus, elderberry, papaya and lemon et al. We then chugged down an E-Z Tea whose ingredients are wolf-berry, ginger, prickly ash, buck thorn bark, blessed thistle, carob and mint.

If you're a vegan ice-cream lover, and who isn't, you must taste David's Butterscotch ice-cream, which is made from raw apricots. It's an elixir, and a delight. Yes David is an alchemist of food. It's easy to see why he's the diet guru of Donna Karen and other celebrities who have gone raw. David's food is not only energizing, it's life-giving and soul-satisfying.

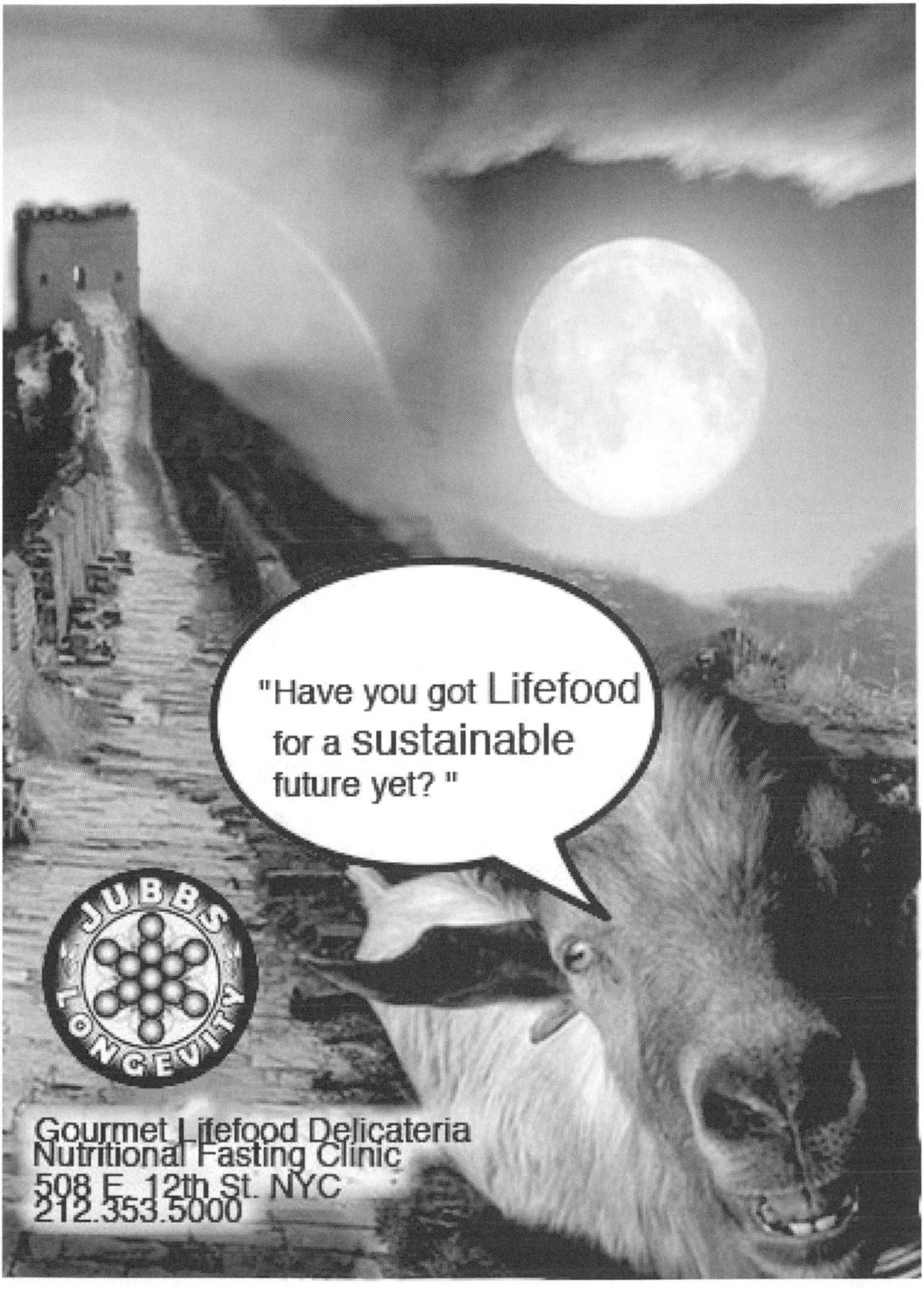
"Have you got Lifefood
for a sustainable
future yet? "
JUBBS LONGEVITY
Gourmet Lifefood Delicateria
Nutritional Fasting Clinic
508 E. 12th St. NYC
212.353.5000

KATE'S JOINT [v] $$ 👍

Full Service
American faux fifties diner style
AE, MC,V
Beer & wine

58 Avenue B
bet. 4th / 5th Streets
212-777-7059
Su-W 8:30 am-11pm
Th-Sa 8am-12pm

Eating at Kate's Joint is like stepping into a Norman Rockwell painting from the fifties. The food as well as the atmosphere are faux fifties--a time when restaurants were called "joints", coffee was called "java," and music poured from the juke box. The food, unlike the food of the fifties, is healthy vegan and vegetarian. Some of the dishes are take-offs on the diner food of the fifties that tasted so good, but was so bad for you. Dishes like Fake Steak, Mock Shepherd's Pie with Salad, Southern Fried Tofu, and Apple Crumb Cake conjure up the fifties originals without inducing a coronary on the way home. [Vegans should be cautious when ordering any dish that contain mock cheese; they may contain casein. Ask the chef.] This is a great place to take your non-veg. friends to coax them off meat, but it's a positive pleasure for anyone. As a chef Kate is great. She and her sister do all the cooking and baking on the premises. Their American home-style dishes are highly original and very tasty. In keeping with the trend towards rawfood eating among vegans and vegetarians, Kate is now offering an organic living-foods menu.

KENOSHA [v] $

Counter service
Midwestern American & South Indian
No cards
No alcohol

543 East Twelfth Street
bet. Avenues A/ B
212-945-8053
daily 11am-11pm

Kenosha is the name of a small town in Wisconsin, which is famous for being the birthplace of the great film director and actor Orson Welles. It's also noted for being the cradle for radio announcers, who were recruited for the country's airwaves because they grew up speaking unaccented Midwestern English. So what's a nice town like Kenosha doing in a place like this? Well, one of the owners is from Kenosha, and he was nostalgic for his hometown. The other owner is Kumi Kulantri of Mumbai, the Indian restaurateur, who has had at least half a dozen restaurants--Dosaria, Thali, Tiffin, et al., shot out from under him. Together they form one of the New York restaurant scene's oddest couples. Their fare is a combination of Midwestern America meets upper middle class Mumbai. We tried their Mango Soup, which is really, really good, and their Veggie Burgers, which were made with colorful shredded vegetables. Kumi made us some delicious Soy Milk Mango Lassis for dessert. We told them that to complete the decor they should put some pictures of Orson Welles on the wall.
•As of this writing, 2008, we are waiting impatiently for Kumi to open Kenosha.

LAN CAFE [v] $ 👍

Full service	342 East 6th Street
Vietnamese	bet. 1st/ 2nd Avenue
No cards	212-228-8325
Beer & wine	daily 11am-10pm

Last summer, we sampled vegan dishes in some Vietnamese restaurants in Hawaii--where there is a large settlement of Vietnamese folk, but, alas, no vegan Vietnamese restaurants. Admittedly, the food was very good, but the food at Lan Cafe--New York's first vegan Vietnamese restaurant--surpasses that of the best in Honolulu. Perhaps it's because the co-owner/chef --Cao Ky and his wife Lan--are devout Mahayana Buddhists and therefore are ethical vegans. Hence, the food is 100% cruelty-free , and, on our many visits, the pure, unalloyed flavors of this essentially Buddhist Vietnamese cuisine shone forth.

In fact, the food at Lan Cafe is so exquisite, that we played a little parlor game--we challenged each other to find a dish on the menu that we didn't like. After repeated visits, we exhausted the menu without being able to find a dish that we didn't adore. All are extraordinary. At Lan Cafe, we must speak of the extraordinary among extraordinaries. These are the best vegan eats of the East!

We recommend that you start with the classic Vietnamese dish --a staple on the menus of restaurants in Saigon--Green Papaya Salad with Mock Shrimp. Follow this with Pho--another classic Vietnamese dish. A capacious bowl is filled with a healthy serving of vegetable broth aswim with long rice noodles, and vegetarian beef. On the side are served bean sprouts and basil leaves. At intervals, these are to be added to the Pho. The flavors, of both the Green Papaya Salad and the Pho, were stupendous!

Fact is: Frank, the manager, had warned us that the Pho at Lan Cafe is so filling that there is scant room for anything else. He was right. We wanted to try the Curried Lemon Grass Seitan, and the Baguettes with Vegetarian Sausage and the one with Vegetarian Mock Ham (an incongruous Gallicism here that is doubtless the legacy of the French colonial occupation of Vietnam)--but we had to postpone those gustatory sensations for our next visit. Our only puzzlement was why was it so easy to find a table here? By rights, there should be lines of vegan gourmets winding around the block.

How did the Lan Cafe get its name. In Vietnamese the word "lan" means "orchid." "Orchidaceous" would aptly describe the cuisine--exotic, eye-filling, and drop-dead delicious!

Doug Green's LIQUITERIA [v] $ 👍

	170 Second Avenue
Counter service	at 11th Street
Natural organic	212-358-0300
V, MC	Winter 7:30am-9pm
No alcohol	Summer 7:30am-11pm

If awards were given for the most hygienic eating establishment in town, Doug Green's Liquiteria would win it hands down. Unlike most juice bar-cum-cafes that have flyblown walls and grimy equipment, Liquiteria has gleaming tiled walls and juicers that are kept spotlessly clean. Every twenty-four hours the juicers are rotated, and disassembled, their parts bathed overnight in a biodegradable sanitizing solution. Floors and walls are scoured at the end of the day. Working surfaces are constantly being wiped down and cleaned. Fruits and vegetables are peeled and scrubbed.

Whereas most juice bars cut corners by using fruit concentrate and non-organic fruit, Doug uses only fresh ingredients and organic fruit whenever possible. And the fruit of all these labors are the most vivid-tasting, health-giving juices and smoothies in the universe. Have the Power Pina Colada Smoothie--banana strawberries, pineapple, organic apple juice. (Skip the bee pollen if you're a vegan). Or try one of Doug's Freshly-Pressed Juices. Extracted using a Norwallk hydraulic press, the most efficient juicer on the market, these juices are said to contain up to five times the minerals, vitamins and enzymes of jus ordinaire.

Try the Grasshopper, one of Doug's hydraulicaly-pressed green juices. It contains organic Hawaian pineapple, organic ginger, organic wheat grass, pears, apples, and mint. Quaff it, and you'll feel like chirping with the crickets.

Heir to a vending machine business, Doug has such a passion for his work that he gave up his family business to "juice the Apple," as he phrases it. A handsome hunk of a guy, Doug--who played football two decades ago at Syracuse--is the best advertisement for the high quality of his product. (He not only owns Liquiteria but he's also its best client.)

Liquiteria enjoys the distinction of being the longest-running, free-standing juice bar in NYC. That staying power seems to have rubbed off on his workers. In an industry with high employee turnover, Doug's polite, hard-working staff have served an average of six years on the job.

Despite its name, Liquiteria doesn't reduce every solid to its liquid state. It's more than a juice bar, it's a place where one may sit down to some of the tastiest soups, salads, wraps, and sandwiches in the land. Many people start their day here with Organic Oatmeal or Organic Granola served with fresh fruit, and organic tea and organic estate grown coffee. Not a few customers are so regular as to take three meals a day here.

Recently Doug hired a special chef to make vegan sushi and salads for their thriving take-out business.

Try the TLT--tempeh-bacon, red leaf lettuce, tomato and soy mayonnaise served on organic 7-grain bread. Or try that old standby, the Peanut Butter and Jelly Sandwich. Doug makes it with fresh-ground Valencia peanuts, layered with a homemade fruit spread, sliced apples and bananas. Sacre bleu! *C'est si deliceuse!*

MADRAS CAFE |v| *$$*

Full service
South Indian, kosher
All major cards

79 Second Avenue
bet. 4th / 5th Streets
212-254-8002
daily 12pm-3pm; 5pm-11pm

Kosher wine & beer

This is the only Indian restaurant in Manhattan that is truly vegan friendly. Eighty percent of the dishes on the menu are vegan, and the ones that are not are explicitly labeled "D" for dairy. The chef-owner, Sridhar Rathnam, is willing to convert any non-vegan dish on the menu to a vegan one. His is also one of the first Indian vegetarian restaurants to use TVP and other soy products in lieu of meat and dairy. Mr. Rathnam told me that he learned the recipes that he uses in the restaurant from his south Indian mother, which explains why the dishes have a down-home flavor. Unusual in an Indian eatery, the vegetables are not overly cooked and are lightly spiced. The dosas and breads are not oily, and even the deep-fried pakoras seem innocent of the oil they were cooked in. Many of our fellow diners were students and instructors from the nearby Jivamukti Yoga Center who drop in after classes. Our favorite dish was the Madras Curried Soy Chunks. But we are also partial to the Vegetable Briyani, and the Stuffed Potato Malbari (a jumbo steamed potato, stuffed with green pea masala, and simmered in traditional Kerala-style coconut curry sauce). When the restaurant, Guru, closed its doors two years ago, Mr. Rathman hired one of its most talented chefs, a lady chef from Kerala. whose work in the kitchen helped elevate the level of the cuisine at Madras Cafe to stratospheric heights. For our money, it is now New York's finest Indian vegetarian restaurant.

MAOZ |v| $

Counter service
Israeli falafel shack, kosher
All Cards
No alcohol
www.maozusa.com

59 East 8th Street
bet. Broadway/ University Place
212-420-5999
daily 11am-12am

See description under Midtown East and other location under Upper West Side.

POMMES FRITES |v| $

123 Second Avenue
Counter Service
bet. Seventh/ Eighth Streets
Belgian French fries
212-674-1234
No cards
daily 11:30am-Midnight
No alcohol

Studies have shown that people go to burger joints mainly for the French fries. With the opening of Pommes Frites and its opposite number, B. Frites at 1657 Broadway, it's now possible for vegetarians to dine on French Fries without having to make a clandestine visit to the Golden Arches. In Belgium, the *maison de pommes frites* is a thriving concern. So some enterprising Americans have imported the idea to New York and judging from the lines that form up at Pommes Frites and B. Frites, it's really taking hold. The fries at Pommes Frites are double cooked in the Belgian manner, and are served with a range of tasty sauces. For vegans, it's necessary to inquire about the composition of the sauces as some may contain mayonnaise and other objectionable ingredients. We managed quite nicely with a double cone of fries that we dipped alternately in etchup and mustard, which are on the house; the other sauces are fifty cents extra.

PUKK [v] **$$**

Full service
Thai vegetarian
All cards
Beer, wine, champagne
www.pukknyc.com

75 First Avenue
bet. 4th/ 5th Streets
212-253-2741
daily 11:30am-11pm

A four-letter word in Thai that means "vegetable," Pukk is an apt name for this all-vegetarian Thai restaurant. Imaginatively designed to make maximum use of the rather cramped dining spaces, Pukk is a model of elegant compression. But the menu enables one to dine spaciously on delicious Thai vegetarian fare. It's not quite vegan here because, inexplicably they serve eggs?!!!? So vegans should inquire about eggs in the noodles, in the pastries, in the soups, and sauces, etc. But everything else is impeccably plant-based. In fact, the Pukksters thoughtfully provide soy milk for tea, coffee, and smoothies. For starters, try the Tom Yum Soup, a yummy soup that is aswim with chunks of spiced tofu, mushrooms, scallions and cilantro; then try the Curry Thai Pancake, a flaky crepe served in a piquant curry sauce. Follow this with the Faux Salmon; or, if you prefer to avoid faux meats, try the tofu dishes--such as Stuffed Tofu, or the Son-in-Law Tofu--at which Thai chefs excel. If there is a rawfooder in your midst, then he or she will be certain to enjoy the All Green Salad, which layers fresh vegetables on a mound of fresh greens. It is nattily and nuttily dressed with a splash of spicy peanut sauce.

Dessert here is a bit of an anticlimax after the crescendo of flavors leading up to it. So we recommend ambling over to Caravan of Dreams, or Babycakes for a truly scrumptious dessert.

Although the food here is not so good as that of the Thai vegan restaurant in Montreal called Chu Chai, which for our money is the best vegan restaurant in the world, it is good enough, because of its sheer exoticism, to be one of the better vegetarian restaurants in New York.

QUINTESSENCE [ve] **$$$** 👍

Full Service
Raw food vegetarian
All cards
No alcohol
www.raw-q.com

263 East 10th Street
bet. 1st Avenue/ Avenue A
646-654-1823
daily 11:am-11pm

For skeptics who think that raw food is a penitential diet of roots, shoots and fruits, Tolentin and her business partner Dan Hoyt, who have been strict rawfoodists for four years, are on a mission to show people that rawfood can be as toothsome as it is nutritious. So admirably have they succeeded that you'd swear that some of the dishes are cooked. Ironically, the mark of a good raw food dish is that it tastes as if it's been cooked. This is certainly true of the Sun Burger, a hearty patty made of sunflower and flaxseed meal mixed with chopped celery, onions, red pepper and herbs dehydrated to a burger consistency and served between slices of dehydrated bread. {The temperature of the dehydrator in which the breads are baked must never rise above an enzyme-killing 120 degrees). Another entree, the Caribbean Nut Meatballs which are served

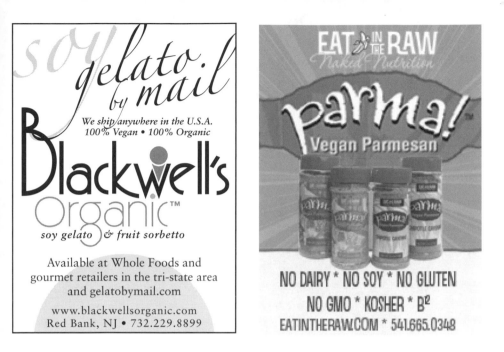
in an aromatic, zesty pineapple-tomato sauce also earns the accolade: "Tastes as if it's been cooked." The Coconut Cream Pie and the Pecan Pie are the quintessence of desserts, fired or unfired, anywhere in the city.

• We were gratified to learn that Quintessence is now 100 percent organic and vegan. When they first opened, we lobbied for them to stop using honey in their dishes, and we like to think that we have played a small role in their going completely vegan. Credit to chef Dan!

WHOLE EARTH BAKERY & KITCHEN [ve] $

Buffet (take-out only)
Organic vegan bakery
No cards
No alcohol

130 St. Marks Place
bet. First Ave/Avenue A
212-677-7597
Su-Th 9am-12am
F-Sa 9am-1am

Hole-in-the-wall offering organic baked goods and small buffet, wholly vegan. The owner assures me that no honey or refined sugar is used. Cheeseless pizza, tofu vegetable turnovers, cabbage knishes, soups and puddings along with whole grain baked goodies of the 100% whole wheat, rather dry variety. For take out mainly — seats four.

SOHO
(Canal Street to Houston Street)

BABYCAKES [ve] **$** 👍

Counter service	248 Broome Street
Vegan baked goods	bet. Orchard/ Ludlow Streets
All cards	212-677-5047
No alcohol	Tu-Th 10am-10pm
www.babycakesnyc.com	F 10am-10pm
	Su-M 10am-8pm

Although the art-deco, retro interior evokes a roadside diner from the 1920's, unless you're a dessertatarian--as we are--then it's not really possible to have a meal here; however, if you have an overdeveloped sweet tooth--as we do--then you could have a chocolate chip cookie as an appetizer, a carrot cupcake as a main course with some extra frosting on the side [It's $1.00 for a side order of frosting.]--and a slice of pound cake for dessert. You could wash it down with a cup of shade-grown, fair-trade Gorilla coffee, as we did.

Here's a rich irony--the owner, Erin McKenna, is an ovo- lacto-vegetarian, but she is scrupulous about not using eggs, or dairy. Instead of honey, she uses stevia and agave nectar -- whereas, the techno-pop star Moby, who is a militant vegan, serves eggs, honey and dairy products at his restaurant, Teany, which is only a few blocks away.

Let's face it, there are a lot of excellent vegan and vegetarian restaurants in New York that have execrable desserts--Pukk, Madras Cafe, Vegetarian Dim Sum House, to list but a few. So, have your dinner at Madras Cafe; then saunter over to Babycakes for some sweet, sweet babycakes for dessert.

PUNJAB [v] **$**

Counter service	114 East First Street
Indian fast food	at Avenue A
No cards	212-533-9048
No alcohol	daily 24 hours

This unprepossessing samosa shack is hard to find, but worth a look-in. It's located in the basement of a building on East First Street with an awning that is misleadingly labeled as a deli-grocery. Down the stairs, one spies Indian cabdrivers munching on samosas, rotis and other vegetarian delights. We mimicked them and ordered a Tikki (potato pancake) slathered with chickpeas and told the counterman that we wanted it without milk, cheese or ghee. Like everyone else in this bustling, cramped place--we ate it standing up. It went down very well.

In the refrigerated display case, there are other pre-cooked curry dishes that just need to be heated in the microwave to be revived. We tried the Curried Bitter Melon, and found it astringent but tasty. The fact that cabbies eat here is a good sign. Typically, cabbies seek out the most flavorful and frugal vegetarian food. So their presence is almost a guarantee of a satisfying meal, however hurried.

TEANY [v] $

	90 Rivington Street
Full service	bet. Orchard/ Ludlow
International	212-475-9190
All cards)	W, Th, Su 10am-10pm
Beer & wine	F, Sa 10am-2am

Teany is a restaurant-cum-teahouse that was founded by the rock star Moby. Its name, Teany, stands for Tea New York, but it is also a pun, referring wryly to its diminutive size. It's teeny as well as teany.

The portions, however, are ample. For instance the faux turkey club sandwich, which we adored, is big enough to feed two people; and the salads, the crostini, and the granola dishes are as generous as they are delicious. Along with the Club Sandwich, we recommend the Crostini. Thin toast ovals are served with four vegan spreads--Olive, White Bean, Artichoke and Herbed Soy Cheese. It's big of Teany that after you've dipped all your toast ovals in the pots of vegan spreads, Teany will freely replenish them.

Teany desserts are tremendous! We particularly liked the Tofu Chocolate Cheese Cake, and the Peanut Butter Chocolate cake, which are supplied to Teany by the Vegan Treats bakery. The eponymous tea menu is as extensive as any four star restaurant's wine list. Last time we were there, we savored the black tea called Golden Monkey,. but there are uncaffeinated herb teas as well. Sad to report: we found the homemade sodas to be flavorless and insipid.

Although Moby is co-owner of the restaurant with his ex-girlfriend Kelly Tisdale, he likens himself to a Victorian father who sees the baby only now and then. He writes the checks but Kelly does the day-to-day running of the shop. In providing such delicious fare in such a tastefully designed space, however teeny--Moby has done the community a whale of a service. Incidentally, Moby, (nee Richard Melvile Hall), is nicknamed after the whale in his distant ancestor, Herman Melvile's novel Moby Dick. He is a committed vegan; one could only wish that he had extended his veganism to the entire menu. Vegan dishes are marked with an asterisk.

TIEN GARDEN [ve] $$ 👍

	170 Allen Street
Full service	at E. Houston/ 1st Avenue
Chinese Homestyle	212-388-1364

All cards   M-Sa 12pm-10pm
No alcohol

Not so long ago, Tiengarden was a lonely outpost of veganism on the lower East Side. Now it may be seen as something of a neighborhood trendsetter. Within the past two years it has become surrounded by eco-conscious stores like Earth Matters and Bluestockings; tony vegan boutiques like MooShoes, and Organic Avenue; and fashionable vegetarian restaurants like Teany.

Based on the ancient theory of five elements--metal, water, earth, and fire--the food at Tiengarden is prepared in such a way as to maximize its chi, or life force. On the other hand, foods that are considered to be sapping of one's chi are scrupulously avoided. So in addition to being vegan, (because animal products are considered to be deleterious to one's chi); the dishes contain no garlic, or onions, which are also held to be harmful to one's chi. Nonetheless, the food is quite delectable without these flavor intensifiers.

We are partial to their Pan-Fried Bean Curd Sandwich, their Mixed Gluten Salad (Spicy braised wheat gluten is served on a bed of lettuce with tomato, celery and carrot sticks and served with a vegan barbecue sauce or vegan mayo.); their Special Nuggets (soy nuggets, red bell peppers, broccoli, cauliflower, zucchini, cashews in a light curry peanut sauce). We also ate with gusto their Basil Beancurd (crisp, layered beancurd with broccoli, tomato and mushrooms in basil sauce).

Unlike most Chinese restaurants, desserts here are totally vegan, substantial, and delicious.,Our current favorite is the Banana Surpise(Fresh bananas surround generous glops of soy ice-cream.) And, like the rest of the food, even their home-made fresh pies and cakes are chi-enhancing.

WILD GINGER [v] **$$** 👍

                                                       380 Broome Street
Full service   bet. Mott/ Mulberry Streets
Pan-Asian   212-966-1883/ 2669
All cards   daily 12pm-11pm
Beer, wine & sake
www. wildgingernyc.com

Three friends--Richard, (the architect and co-manager), Winnie (the accountant and manager), and her husband, Tim (the chef)--have pooled their assets, as it were, to create one of the most popular and successful vegetarian restaurants in town. Richard is responsible for the elegant yet cozy interior; Winnie, for the crisply efficient running of the place; and Tim for the tasty dishes. "Pan Asian" is how they describe their cuisine--Thai, Chinese, Malaysian and Indian--and for once the menu truly deserves this overused and often inaccurate appellation.

We practically shouted our adulation of the Scallion Pancakes with the Home-Made Mango Salsa, which tasted less like crepes than small pizzas topped with a piquant mango sauce. We adored the Samosa in Curry Sauce. Their newest appetizer, Tempeh in Satay Sauce is supernal. For the main course, our taste buds thrilled to the exotic flavor notes in Malaysian

Curry Stew (Mild, Slow-Cooked Coconut Curry with Soy Protein, Broccoli, Carrots, Potatoes and Pumpkin). and Mango Soy Protein (Thin-Slice Medallions Sautéed in a Mellow Plum Sauce with Mango, Zucchini, Sweet-Sage Turnips, Peppers, and Onions).

Beverages--we tossed off the homemade Wild Ginger Beer, and Virgin Mojitoes with gusto. They were--at least to our teetotal, non-alcoholic sensibilities-- bewitching. For drinkers of more adult beverages, there is an array of beers, wine and sakes that are guaranteed to "bewitch, bother and bewilder." Vegans, however, should beware the Lassis (an Indian drink made with fruit juice and yogurt). Order soy-milk Lassis instead!

Chef Tim accrued his repertoire of Pan-Asian vegan dishes by working in a string of different veg. restaurants--such as Zen Palate, Tien Garden and assorted others--as a sous-chef. But by now, Tim has clearly outstripped his masters; so while one may recognize many of the menu dishes from having dined elsewhere, seldom have they been prepared to such palate-pleasing perfection.

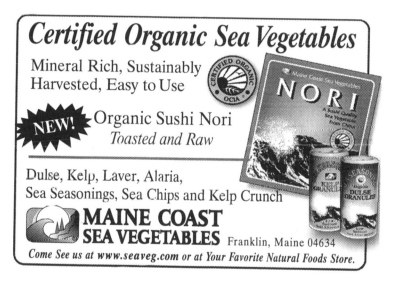

BELOW CANAL STREET
(Includes Chinatown, Tribeca, Financial District)

BUDDHA BODAI VEGETARIAN RESTAURANT [v] **$$**

Full service
Chinese (kosher)
All cards
No alcohol.

5 Mott Street
at Bowery
212-566-8388
daily 10:30am-10:30pm

See description under Queens

HOUSE OF VEGETARIAN |v| **$** 👍

Full service
Chinese Homestyle
No cards
11pm
Beer & wine

68 Mott Street
bet. Canal/Bayard Streets
212-226-6572
daily 11am

This is one Chinatown restaurant where there aren't any fresh kills hanging in the window. "All We Are Served Vegetarian Dishes" reads the reassuring note on the extensive menu of more than 200 dishes, from Vegetarian Roast Duck (too much of a poultry flavor for our taste) to Braised Chicken with Lily Flowers (made from wheat gluten) or everybody's favorite, Iron Steak, made from yams and quite tasty. Our own personal favorite were mock Chicken with Mango and Black Mushrooms With Soysticks. Served in a narrow dining room with plastic tablecloths and no ambiance, but the food's good and there's plenty of it.

LITTLE LAD'S BASKET |v| **$** 👍

Self service, buffet
International
No cards
No alcohol

120 Broadway
Concourse level
212-227-5744
Bkfst M-F 7:30am-10:30am
Lunch 11am-3pm

Like Dr. John "Cornflakes" Kellogg, Larry, the owner of Little Lad's is a 7th-Day Adventist, who is on a mission to convert the world to vegetarianism one-meal at a time. However, he makes it plain that he is not funded by the Adventist Church. They encourage him but they don't provide him with any financial backing.[Did we detect a trace of acrimony in his admission?]

Larry has used the same formula in creating the Little Lad's chain--{He envisages it as a globe-girdling chain of vegetarian restaurant franchises.)--that he used in his previous restaurant venture--Country Life, which was a veg.restaurant chain that once girdled the US and Europe in the early 1990's. Successful, though it was, it failed from exuberant over-expansion. It was wildly popular during its heyday in New York and Boston. People still remember it wistfully.

We had a vegan mock Shepherd's Pie, a vegan French Onion Soup, and a Cheeseless Cheese Cake. All delicious and all for only $3.99.Larry, who mans the register, took our money. Judging from the high quality and low price of the food here, Little Lad's will be around at least until the Second Advent.

VEGETARIAN DIM SUM HOUSE [ve] $$ 👍

	24 Pell Street
Full service	at Mott Street
Chinese	212-577-7176
No cards	daily 11am-11pm
No alcohol	

Vegetarian Dim Sum House serves most of the same dishes that its sister restaurant, House of Vegetarian, serves except that it offers them amid posher surroundings with a wider range of dim sum dishes. "Dim Sum" (literally "cooked snacks") are the snack-like dishes that are popular in Hong Kong, Taiwan and other parts of South China. The Cantonese like to put together several dim sum dishes for breakfast, lunch and tea; they even have a few dim sum dishes as appetizers before dinner. Because they may eat dim sum three or four times a day, these snacks have to be skillfully prepared to avoid boring the jaded palate. The dim sum that we had at the Dim Sum House were certainly unboring. We particularly liked the Spinach Dumpling, the Lotus Root Cake, and the Sticky Rice wrapped in Lotus Leaf. From the main course menu, we liked the mock roast duck and the mock chicken dishes made from tofu skin. Portions are generous and service is attentive.

ZEN PALATE [ve] $$ 👍

	663 Ninth Avenue
Full service	at 46th Street
Asian vegetarian	212-582-1669
All major cards	daily 11:30am-10:45pm
No alcohol	

See description under Midtown East.

BROOKLYN

BLISS [v] $$

Full service
Natural
No cards
No alcohol

Bedford Avenue
bet. N6th / N7th Streets
718-599-2547
daily 8am-11pm

"Bliss was it in that dawn to be alive and eating brunch at Bliss, but to be vegetarian was very heaven!" is what Wordsworth might have written had he been a vegetarian and had he had the good fortune to dine at Bliss--one of New York's better vegetarian restaurants. He would surely have waxed poetic over the vegan BLT's that are made with Fakin' Bacon, the Veggie Burgers and the Seitan "Steak" Sandwiches. The salads are a tone poem and the desserts an ode to Bliss. With prices so much lower in Williamsburg than for comparable fare in Manhattan, it's worth hopping the L train and traveling East just one stop from Manhattan for so much more bliss for the buck.
    • Recent visits, in late 2008, yielded less bliss for the buck, but it's still worth a subway jaunt.

BODY AND SOUL[ve] $

Food stand
International, organic
No cards
No alcohol

Farmers' Market
at Grand Army Plaza
212-982-5870
Sa 8am-4pm
Sa 8am-4pm

One of the best ways to keep body and soul together in the city is to have a light vegan meal at the vegan food stand in the Grand Army Plaza Farmers' market., which is called aptly enough Body and Soul. Started by the owners of Counter restaurant back in 1994, it draws throngs of hungry folk for breakfast, lunch, early light suppers, and snacks. And it's easy to see why. The out-size wraps and turnovers are scrumptious. Try the Saffron Potato wrap which teases the palate with plantain chunks hidden inside. Or try the Spinach Portabello Turnover, which is filled with tofu ricotta, and tastes a bit like a Spinach Lasagna. You might want to complement this with a dairy-free Blueberry Muffin, Or a Sweet Potato Muffin. Don't leave the stand without biting into a melt-in-your-mouth Chocolate Brownie, or a Wheat-Free Almond Cookie. Then repair to one of the benches in Prospect Park and have an *al fresco* meal.

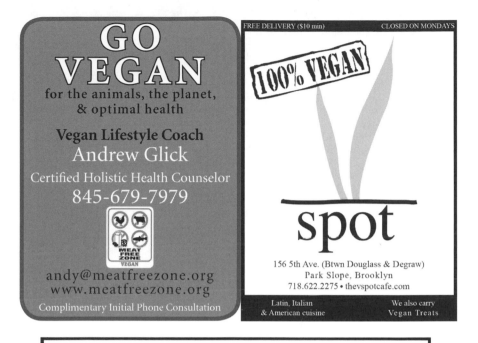
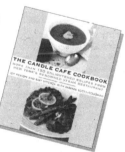
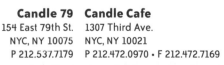

"D" ITAL SHAK [ve] $

Counter service
Trinidadian vegan (no cards)
$5.00-8.00
No alcohol

989 Nostrand Aveune
bet. Empire / Sullivan
718-756-6557
M-Sa 24 hours

According to the Trinidadian family who runs this highly successful vegan eatery, in Trinidadian patois, "D" stands for the article "the." The word "Ital" in Caribbean creole means vegan. The unique feature of this restaurant, which sets it apart from every other vegan establishment in New York City, is that it is open 24 hours a day. So, if you're a Manhattanite and are suddenly seized with a craving for Ackee Patties or Callaloo at two in the morning, then jump on the number two train and get thee to "D" Ital Shak. The most popular dish on the menu is a vegetarian version of macaroni and cheese, which is made with soy cheese. The Sorrel and Mauby drinks are bracing, and the dessert, Plantain Tart, is as sinful as it sounds. The place is always packed, even at two in the morning. (It's so successful, in fact, that the managers said that they didn't need to be mentioned in the Vegan Guide!) So be prepared to stand in line. Your taste buds will thank you.

EARTHTONEZ [v] $

Full service
Organic wraps, sandwiches, desserts
All cards
No alcohol

349 Fifth Avenue
bet. Fourth/ Fifth Streets
718-395-1516
daily 11am-10pm

Two civic-minded fellows, Jumaane Williams and K. Bain, who were best friends at Brooklyn College, dreamed of opening a vegetarian restaurant in Park Slope. They wanted to educate the community about the health and environmental benefits of eating a plant-based diet. To that end, having no experience in the restaurant field, they enrolled in a city sponsored restaurant training workshop, and with the help of Robert Walsh, the head of the Dept of small Business Services, they learned to navigate the city's notorious red tape.

We thoroughly enjoyed their Mock Tuna Salad, which comes in two flavors—Curried Vegan and Middle Eastern Vegan.

We relished the Dub (vegan chicken, smothered in sweet peppers, onions, and spicy jerk sauce). We demolished the Tofurger (home-made tofu patties with sautéed mushrooms and shredded vegan mozzarella, served on a gluten-free bun). For dessert, we abolished the Red Velvet layer cake and the Strawberry Cheesecake. Both desserts were concocted by a supernal Brooklyn vegan bakery named Red Mango. Throughout the meal, we sipped kiwi-berry, and orange-tangerine Switch Sodas made with unsweetened carbonated fruit juice.

Like an urban fairy tale come true, the two friends opened Earth Tonez last December. And, we're here to tell you that their dream was fulfilled. The food is pluperfect!

FOODSWINGS [ve] **$** 👍

295 Grand Street
Counter service
Fast food
All cards
No alcohol

bet. Roebling/ Havemeyer
718-388-1919
T-Th 2pm-11pm;
F 2pm-2am, Sa 12pm-2am;
Su 11am-11pm

The most conscientious fast-food joint on the planet, this has got to be. The owner, Freedom Tripodi, is on a mission to stamp out the addictive, carnivorous fastfoodism that is rampaging through the nation. He is fighting it by providing a tasty range of vegan fast food edibles that surpass even those served at Red Bamboo and Kate's Joint. What's his secret? Perhaps it's that he's added to his food a subtle ingredient--a dash of compassion. For instance, he is emphatic about serving food that is free of dairy products and honey; he donates his food and his services to animal rights organizations. (Recently he catered a Farm Sanctuary Gala gratis.) And, he puts out vegan munchies after 11pm so that the clients of the numerous taverns in the neighborhood will have vegan treats to snack on when they stagger through the door for a postprandial feed.

They're all here--vegan versions of the abominable but addictive foods concocted by Colonel Sizzle-Hop MacWendys. Fish sticks, chicken nuggets, hot dogs, fried shrimp, buffalo wings, hamburgers, cheese burgers, drumsticks, et al. By far the most popular dish (according to Freedom) is the Faux Philly Cheese Steak Sandwich, but we preferred the Tempeh Wrap and the mock No Chicken Parmigiana Sandwich.(breaded chicken cutlets, with soy mozzarella covered in tomato sauce, served on warm Italian bread), and the No Turkey Club, (a double decker sandwich with pepper soy turkey slices, crispy soy bacon, romaine lettuce and tomato) is better than Teany's. It comes with your choice of soy mayo or mustard. We also liked the Foodswings Pu-Pu Platter, which contains 2 Mock Nuggets, 2 Sea Styx, 2 "Shrimp," and 1 each of Foodwings Drumsticks, as well as the sauces that come with each--such as Bleu Cheese, Agave-Mustard, Tartar, BBQ--that are mocked to a fare thee well.

Best of all, are the French Fries, (Freedom Fries?), which put those served by the Golden Arches to shame. [Studies have shown that people go to the Golden Arches and other burger joints mainly for the French Fries.]

Prepared off premises by two companies, Vegan Treats and Miss Vegan Goddess, the desserts here are otherworldly. We especially liked the faux cheesecake, and the Strawberry Cake, but our favorite, was the Key-Lime Pie created by Sarah Sohn, "Miss Vegan Goddess." Eat the food here and you'll feel like a vegan god or goddess just out of your teens.

4 COURSE VEGAN [ve] **$$$** 👍

Williamsburg Loft
(Call for precise location)
718-599-5913
Sa/ Su 7-11pm

Full service
International, organic
$40.00 prix-fixe (no cards)
Organic wine
www.4 course vegan.com

Just ten blocks away from the restaurant Bliss, an even more blissful dining experience awaits you. In a Williamsburg loft, an idealistic ethical vegan, Matteo Silverman, has created an offbeat culinary experience that every New Yorker, veg or non-veg, owes it to his taste buds to partake of. Early in the week, Matteo decide what dishes he's going to feature for the following Saturday, then posts them on his website--www.4coursevegan.com. He also sends out hard copies of the bill of fare to stores like Moo Shoes, where we first learned about them. The menu changes weekly, and one must call or Email to make reservations, and to ask for directions on how to find their loft..

On the night we visited, there were twelve guests, among whom two were vegans, three were ovo-lacto vegetarians, the rest were carnivores. Which made for a lively evening. We sat next to a Belgian artist, a denizen of Williamsburg, whose favorite dish in the world was viand du cheval, a delicacy in Belgium. They even have restaurants dedicated to that detestable dish. So we had a heated discussion on the merits of veganism vs. the demerits of viand du cheval.

That's the great thing about Four Course Vegan. It's a sort of vegan "My Dinner With Andre." But playing verbal tennis with our table mates did not prevent us from savoring each course. We started with Meyer Lemon Aleppo Chile Aioli. This was followed by Creamy Artichoke and Baby Spinach Phyllo Triangles. Then for the piece de la resistance, we were served Spring Vegetable Paella with Spiced Seitan Smoked Tofu, and Saffron Basmati Rice. Dessert was Pecan Tart with Vanilla Bean Ice Cream and Chocolate Chards.

Our most recent in a succession of follow-up visits coincided with 4-Coourse Vegan's 5th anniversary! 4- Course has had more staying power than many a full-time restaurant. With his customary elan, Chef Matteo tossed in a few extra cousrses that night, so the evening ended up being a 7-course affair. We particuarly relshed the watermelon salad (piquent watermelon slices serd ona bd of alfalfa). There isn't a dish that we didn't swoon over. When he's not regaling the guests at 4-course Vegan, Chef Matteo does personal cheffing for celebrities like Kenin Bacon, and Woody Harrelson. In his spare time, Chef Mateo is a food inventor. He's just delvelped a raw vegan dog treat with will soon be on the market, and he's also invnented a vegan raw macaroon, which he will be intoudcing to his Chef Matteo poduct line. It's refreshing to dine out and not have to ask if there's any milk in the soup, casein in the dip, or honey in the dessert. Chef Matteo is such a principled vegan that he won't have these "ingredients" in his kitchen.

FOUR SEASONS RESTAURANT [ve} $

	2281 Church Avenue
Counter service	at Bedford Avenue
Caribbean vegetarian	718-693-7996
$4.00-10.00 [no cards}	M-Th 9am-10pm
No alcohol	Fr-Sa 9am-12; Su 11am-7pm

This is not to be confused with the higher rent, higher cholesterol restaurant of the same name in Manhattan. This is the healthier vegetarian version. It's Fresh Assorted Curries, Vegetarian Lo Mein, Vegan Baked Goods and Fresh-Squeezed Juices will delight your palate and are guaranteed to ward off a thrombosis.

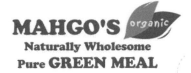

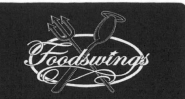

IMHOTEPS [ve] $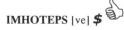

734 Nostrand Ave.
Self service
bet. Park Place & Prospect
West Indian vegetarian, organic
718-493-2395
No cards
daily- 8:30am-12am
No alcohol

Imhoteps is the name of an Egyptian minister during the reign of the pharaoh Zoser, who ruled Egypt about 2650 BCE. Imhotep's wisdom was so vast that he has been deified as the creator of medicine and the epitome of sagacity. The owners of this Brooklyn eatery--Tonde and Maketa-- named both their first son and their restaurant after this legendary Egyptian sage. Had Imhoteps been a chef then he could not have crafted a tastier or a healthier cuisine than the food that is on offer at Imhoteps. The chef Victor Telesford was the founding chef at Veggie Castle, and his skill at the stove did a lot to make Veggie Castle the roaring success that it is today. The food is so seductive that many customers eat three meals a day here. Among the dishes that are especially recommended are Soy Salmon and Vegie Roast Duck, but everything on the menu is mouth-watering. The beverages, which include protein shakes, sorrel, wheat grass and sea-moss juices are healthful and bracing. We had a glass of Sorrel with our Soy Salmon and Veggie Roast Duck and topped off our meal with a Carrot Sea Moss vegan ice cream that was laced with gingko--the memory enhancing herb--that made the whole culinary experience even more unforgettable.

JILL'S [ve] $$

Counter service
231 Court Street
Organic wild crafted foods
bet. Warren/ Baltic Streets
All Cards
718-797-0330
No alcohol
M-Sa 11am-9pm
www.jillpettitjean.com
Su 11am-8pm

Just before it opened, Jill's was being touted everywhere as the newest, modish rawfoods restaurant. So, we were a little taken aback when, one afternoon, we ambled in only to see a chef, standing at the western base of a rectangular counter area, furiously frying up food for Jill's ravenous patrons. Droplets of perspiration were flying off his forehead; his hair was askew; and he didn't have a moment to spare to answer some of our questions about the place.

The menu states that the dishes are "a fusion of raw and kindly cooked foods." How kindly they were cooked is a matter of opinion. In fact, because there's only one harried chef, desperately trying to turn out all the dishes on two little gas rings, we've seldom seen food so aggressively cooked!

That said, the appetizer we tried, Leafy Green Wrap with Spicy Tamarind Dressing, went down very well. The entree that we sampled, Asparagus and Shiitake Mushroom Barley Risotto, was mighty tasty and we hasten to recommend it. Curiously enough, for a quasi-rawfoods restaurant, only two of the entrees were uncooked--a raw Lasagna, and a Reuben Wrap. Albeit, there is a shiny display case with all sorts of raw treats on view.

For dessert, we had a raw cookie, which made us wonder if it might have tasted better had it been aggressively cooked. Nonetheless, we recommend Jill's because it is vegan, because it has generally good-tasting food, and because it just a few blocks south of one of our favorite bookstores in the city, BookCourt. The latter is superbly well stocked, and is without a doubt the best bookstore in Brooklyn. Be sure to stop in for a browse after you've dined at Jill's.

LUCKY CAT, THE [v] $ 👍

Counter service
Paninis and pizza
All cards
Full bar
www.TheLuckyCat.com

245 Grand Street
bet. Roebling/ Driggs
718-782-0437
M-Th 12pm-2am;
F-Sa 10am-4am;
Su 10am-2am

Lucky is the cat who strays into this. the first veg. nightclub in the city! We say, "stray" because the owners of Lucky Cat have done little to publicize the fact that they are a veg. nightclub. So, most of the customers wander in, not knowing that the owners, Lilah and Sascha, are vegetarians and that the chef is vegetarian. Nor do their customers suspect that with its use of compostable utensils made from corn and sugar cane—Lucky Cat is impeccably green! It's high time that it stop being such a well- kept secret. Especially, as the pizzas here are formidable! [As are the paninis and the seasonal salads.]

The chef, who tells us that he has been making oven-baked pizza for the past twelve years is only twenty-seven. That means he started baking pies at fifteen. And his experience shows in the texture and flavor of the pizzas that we devoured. We had two ten-inch personal pizzas--The Vegan (tomato sauce, spinach, chili flakes, herbed tomatoes, and truffle oil); The Con Mojos (grilled eggplant and zucchini, fresh garlic and red and green mojos), Pluperfect!

This is the place to come if you're a vegan pining for cheeseless pizza. The chef doesn't care to use ersatz cheese. Rather, he prefers just to serve it, naked of cheese, but with piquant veggie toppings like grilled eggplant.

We munched our pizzas in the gazebo in the backyard, where we were dismayed to see that there is a sunken aquarium, crammed with carp and goldfish, who were obviously agitated by the lack of space and the charivari. Then we re-entered the club, where a live music act was in full swing. So we sipped two vegan smoothies--a Johnny's Compromise (banana, strawberries, cream of coconut, pineapple juice, sprinkled cinnamon)--and--so we could stay up late and vibrate to the music--an All Nighter (espresso, banana, soymilk and hazelnut).

MIGHTY DIAMOND [v] $

Self service
Caribbean style, vegetarian
All cards
No alcohol

347 Graham Avenue
bet Metropolitan/ Conselyea
718-384-7778
daily- 12pm-11pm

Named after the famous Jamaican Reggae band, Mighty Diamond, this restaurant is owned and managed by Laura and her partner Gregg, neither of whom is African-American, Jamaican, Rastafarian, or vegan. Much as the entrees here are ersatz meat, the restaurant--right down to the pastel murals depicting the Lion of Judah, and the hand of fate on the walls-- is ersatz Rasta.

Although not even a lacto-vegetarian Laura told us that she became enamored of Rastafarian food, when she lived near the late, lamented Veggie Castle, which served real Rasta vegan food. [They've since relocated to Queens.] She spent some years collecting recipes and studying Rasta cooking techniques during several forays to Jamaica.

The upshot of it is: She and her partner started this pseudo-Rasta, almost-vegan restaurant--she confided to us with tongue in cheek—in order to have a healthful place to eat-- and partly to do penance for owning a riotously successful saloon down the street.

We, as fussy vegans declined to try their star dish, which is Jerk Tofu because it was made with honey, but we did try the Curry "Goat," which is made with seitan and potatoes and Rasta condiments. We also liked their Garlic Collard Greens, and Quinoa. The Esco-"Fish," which is their version of the Caribbean staple, Escovitch Fish, was less successful. The Mango Nectar and Iced Hibiscus Tea, that we guzzled with our food, were most refreshing.

As a Rastafarian restaurant, Mighty Diamond falls short. But as an almost-vegan restaurant that serves some mighty tasty dishes, the Mighty Diamond is culinary curio that it worth a look-in.

PERELANDRA [v] $ 👍

Counter service
Internatinal
All Cards
No alcohol
www. perelandra natural.com

175 Remsen Street
bet. Court/ Clinton
718-855-6068
M-F 8:30-8:30
Sa 9:30-8:30:
Su 11-7

On their way to work, Brooklyn's pinstripe brigade pauses here just long enough to scarf down the Breakfast Sandwich, which is Perelandra's answer to the ghastly EggMaguffin (sic.). The Perelandra version consists of baked tofu, tempeh bacon, avocado, dill, and caramelized onion served on a Freshly Baked Spelt Muffin. Yummmy! Organic oatmeal with a different fresh fruit is served daily.

The pinstriped set returns for lunch, and it is not uncommon to see a long line of men and women in business suits standing politely in a line that insinuates itself through the store (Brooklyn's largest health food store). With courts and investment houses hard by, we are in Brooklyn's legal and business district. Eaten up with curiosity, we eavesdropped on the line-waters'c onversations: Sure enough, torts as well as tortes were being hotly discussed.

Every day Perelandra's menu changes, but the categories remain the same. For instance, every day they offer a Soup; a Sauce and Grain, A Casserole a Sandwich: a Wrap; an Entree and a Dessert.

For lunch we slurped their fresh Miso Soup; then savored the Japanese Wasabi Potato Salad and a Barbecue Un-Chicken Sandwich. We also sampled their Baked Vegetable Risotto. For the grand finale, we downed their inimitable Tofu Vegan Cheesecake. For the post prandial

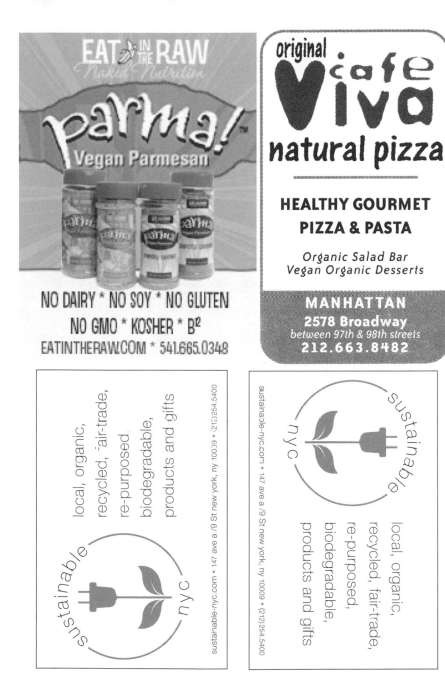

beverage, we sipped their Avocado Smoothie. Which contains Coconut Juice, Avocado, Agave Nectar, and Fresh Lime Juice. We specifically requested that they make it with Agave nectar as they ordinarily make it with honey. After the ethical sweetener were added, we tossed it off with gusto! Replete with delilcous vegan food and drink, we wobbled through the store's portal into a sun-splashed Brroklyn summer afteroon.

RAW STAR [v] $$

Counter service	687 Washington Avenue
Raw West Indian Cuisine	bet. St. Marks/ Prospect
No Cards	718-975-0304
No alcohol	Tu-Sa 11am-11pm
wwwrawstarcafe.com	Su 9am-11pm

The newest star in the firmament of rawfood restaurants is Mawule Job Simon's Raw Star. The décor is reminiscent of Mawule's ill-starred venture, Green Paradise, which opened iin 2003, but went kaput in 2004 because it was too far ahead of its time. From Green Paradise, Mawule has salvaged the counter made from palm wood and thatched palm fronds, which he built by himself (proving that he is as handy with a hammer and saw as he is with a spatula). The chartreuse walls are festooned with works of art, the most striking of which s a painting depicting scantily clad rawfoodists frolicking in an African Eden. The background music consists of reggae versions of popular tunes--to the strains of which we ate our sumptuous meal.

A native of Trinidad, Mawule, earned his stripes as a raw chef by training at Brooklyn's now defunct SunFire juice Club with the legendary Aris La Tham, America's first vegan rawfood gourmet chef.

Aris has since decamped to Jamaica where he runs a Sunfired Spa in Ochos Rios. The best way to taste Aris' food without traveling to Ocho Rios is to eat at Raw Star. Mawule pays homage to his mentor by including a few of Aris's signature dishes on the menu. Such s Tree Fruit, Curried Plantain, Tain. Whis Salad and the ineffable Banana Cream Pie.

But Mawule is an innovative rawfood chef in is own right. He adds a Trinidadian fillip to the dishes that delight and deceive the palate.

Many of his dishes are *trompe l'oeil* for the tongue. For instance, his raw Tabouleh is actually made with cauliflower florets that are prepared to look like grains of cracked wheat. Similarly, he makes a raw tempeh dish which really isn't tempeh, but is made from a variety of unfired vegetables. The artfully prepared dishes tease and titillate the palate. The dessert, which pays tribute to the master, Aris La Tham, that we favored is his raw Banana Cream Pie. Its flavor notes along with those of almost every other dish on the menu at Raw Star are positively celestial.

RED BAMBOO [v] $$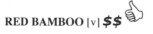

271 Adelphi Street
at DeKalb Avenue
718-643-4352
Tu-F 12pm-12am
Sa-Su 11am-12am

Full service
Asian soul food fusion
$9.95-12.95 (all cards)
No alcohol
www.redbamboobrooklyn.com

See description under Greenwich Village

'sNICE [v] $

45 8th Avenue
at 3rd Street
718-788-2121
daily 7:30am-10pm

Self service
Sandwiches, salads, baked goods
All cards
Beer & wine

See description under Greenwich Village

STRICTLY VEGETARIAN [ve] $

2268 Church Avenue
bet.Bedford/Flatbush Avenues
718-284-2543
daily noon-11:30pm

Counter service
Carribean vegetarian
$4.00-8.00 (no cards)
No alcohol

Just down the street from the late Veggie Castle with which it can stand comparison, this place serves such delicious Caribbean vegetarian dishes as Chick Pea Stew, Vegetable Chow Mein and Tofu Stew. The menu changes daily.

URBAN SPRING [v] $

185 DeKalb Avenue
at Carlton
718-237-0797
daily 8am-7:30pm

Full service
Internatinal
Cash only
No alcohol
www. Urbanspring.net

If trophies were handed out for the greenest vegetarian restaurant, then Gordon and his wife Consuela—owners of Urban Spring—would win in a walk. This cozy eatery in Brooklyn's tony Fort Green section is furnished and decorated with building materials reclaimed from a condemned church in Washington Square—the Peace church. [The church's first bishop, Matthew Simpson encouraged Abraham Lincoln to denounce slavery. He eulogized Lincoln at his funeral.] It's rather poignant that this historic church survives only in the parts that have been rescued by Urban Spring.

The electricity is supplied by wind power. All the utensils, plates, and cups are made from post-consumer corn, potato and sugar cane fibers. If you were really, really hungry, you could eat the utensils! Happily, the food here is so satisfying and delicious, that eating the plates, forks and spoons wouldn't cross your mind.

Two of their sandwiches are much the best we've tasted in a long, long time--Avocado Sprouts & Tangy Lemon Tahini Spread (with cucumber, shredded carrots & optional diced red onion). The other is Tempeh Avocado (with ginger baked tempeh, cilantro, homemade radish pickles, and shredded carrots). In fact we liked them so much that we hereby proclaim them to be the best two sandwiches in all five boroughs.

After downing the sandwiches, we gulped two smoothies—Creamy Coconut Cardomom (blended with homemade Brazil nut milk, dates, bananas, and cardomom); and the Tropi-Cal (fresh cashew milk, dates, bananas, and coconut). We liked that they were made with nut milks instead of soymilk, which is a technique that Gordon admittedly learned from Dr. David Jubb of Jubb's Longevity. Gordon wanted us to mention that Leslie McEachern, proprietor of the inimitable Angelica Kitchen, helped him and his wife to design the menu. She even lent them her chef for a brief space.

For dessert, we savored the Raw Key Lime Pie (with lime, avocado mousse on a cashew coconut crust). The raw pie was assembled on the premises, and the breadstuffs and other baked goods are baked on the premises. We hope Urban Spring springs eternal.

V-SPOT CAFE, THE [ve] $$ 👍

Full service
South American/ Italian vegan
All cards
Beer & wine
thevspotcafe.com

156 Fifth Avenue
bet. Douglass/ Degraw Streets
718-622-2275
T-Th 11am -10:pm
F-Su 11am-11pm
Brunch Sa-Su 11am-4pm

Verily an erogenous zone for the vegan palate is Daniel Carabano's new Park Slope vegan eatery called the "V-spot." Here the dishes are. in the uncensored words of a lady friend, who dines there often--"Sooooo gooood!" We certainly wanted to have what she was having; so we ventured over to the V-Spot to see what all the fuss and bother was about. There in an intimate room, with black-and-white photos of Brooklyn adorning exposed brick walls, we savored the V-Spot experience.

Serious vegans, will be impressed by the V-Spot's dedication to ethical standards. The menu proclaims: "All of our dishes are strictly vegetarian. That is, they do not contain any meat chicken, fish, eggs, milk, cheese, honey, casein, gelatin, whey or any other animal or animal derived product. Our mock meat products are meatless and contain soy." Clearly the V in this V-Spot is not for Vendetta, but for Victory!

Dan, the owner, who often doubles as a waiter, took our order. A high-school math-teacher-turned-vegan restaurateur, Dan is a true Pythagorean. [Pythagoras--as you were probably not instructed in your high school geometry classes--founded a society for the study of mathematics in ancient Greece which required that its initiates be strict vegetarians or vegans.]

Most of the dishes on the menu are based on family recipes--such as the appetizer Empanadas--that Dan inherited from his Colombian paternal grandmother. Even the seemingly prosaic Steak with Rice & Beans (Bandeja Paisa)--is reminiscent of the authentic *comida* to be had in the village cantinas of South America. Its authenticity--albeit veganized,--is why it, and so many of the other dishes with a Latin flair, are so utterly transporting.

The Latin flair extends to Italian specialties such as Lasagna, "Chicken" with Eggplant; Quinoa Pasta Marinara, Eggplant Parmigiana Hero and the Veggie Tacos that danced fandangos on our tongue. Piquant also were the side orders of Spinach with Garlic and Oil; Plantains; Sweet Potato Fries, and Grilled Asparagus. To the latest menu, Dan has added two superb new dishes. An appetizer:Raw Nori Rolls (A ginger almond pate surrounds a center of spinach and carrots) plus a new entree: Tofu Thai Curry. Desserts are the dependably scrumptious vegan treats from Vegan Treats Bakery.

VEGETARIAN PALATE   [v] $$

	258 Flatbush Avenue
Full service	Bet Prospect Park/ St. Marks
Chinese	718-623-8809
All cards	M-Th 11:30am-11pm
No alcohol	Fr, Sa 11:30am, 11:30pm
	Su: 12:00--11:00pm

Vegetarian Palate probably has the most extensive menu of any vegetarian restaurant in the city. Which reminds us of the famous adage that you should never fall in love with someone who has more problems that you, or play cards with someone named "Doc," or eat in a restaurant named "Mom's,"--or in one that has a superabundance of items on the menu. Like most Chinese vegan restaurants Vegetarian Palate abounds in mock meats--as witness their vegetarian seafood dish, Ocean Harvest, which features a collection of vegetarian shrimp, scallops, and squid served with broccoli, snow peas, and baby corn. But the ultimate mock meat tour de force is their Paella Valencia , which is composed of sundry mock seafoods such as shrimp, scallops, crab, mock chicken, mock eel, tofu, shitake mushrooms with mixed vegetables. The service is crisply efficient, the decor, garish. Other diners have complained of excessive starch and oil in the dishes, but one may request of the waiter that these additives be omitted. We had the Soy Chicken with Spinach in Curry Sauce, and the Soy Lemon Chicken and our palates were beguiled by them. For dessert we indulged ourselves in a Banana Split, made with three scoops of non-dairy ice-cream covered with sprinkles and chocolate syrup--all of which soothed our vegetarian palate.

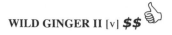

WILD GINGER II [v] **$$**

Full service
Pan-Asian
All cards
Beer, wine & sake
www. wildgingernyc.com

212 Bedford Avenue
at North 5th Street
718-218-8828
Daily 12pm-11pm

For description, see under Soho.

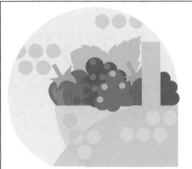

Congratulations:

The Vegan Guide to New York City

On Your 15th Anniversary! Keep Up the Excellent Work!

...Compliments of a Friend

QUEENS

ANNAM BRAHMA [v] $

Full service
Indian vegetarian
$4.00-12.00 (all cards)
No alcohol

84-43 164th Street
at Hillside Avenue
718-523-2600
M-Tu,Th-Sa 11am-10pm
W 11am-4pm; Su 12-10pm

This year marks the thirty-eighth anniversary of Annam Brahma, making it one of the most venerable vegetarian restaurants in the city. It was started and is currently operated by followers of the spiritual leader Sri Chimnoy, who encourages his pupils to observe a vegetarian diet, to meditate and to give something back to the community. (Pictures of Chimnoy running marathons and striking poses festoon the walls). His pupils founded this restaurant to contribute to the common weal; and the high quality of the food bespeaks their dedication to higher principles. Particularly recommended are the delicious Chapati Roll-Ups that are stuffed with either an American Veggie Burger filling or an Indian Curry filling, and the Veggie Kebabs made with soy meat.

BREAD A. CAFE [v] $

Counter service
Chinese-Japanese-American fusion, organic
M, V
No alcohol
www. Breadaorganic.com

41-46 College Point Boulevard
bet. 41st Road/ Sanford
718-886-8828
daily 8:30am-8pm

Brenda Hwang, the proprietor of this cozy little café in Queens is a former fashion designer, an alumna of FIT, who had her own boutique on Fifth Avenue, and a staff of forty people toiling under her. In 2006, she turned her back on her thriving design company, and opened this vegetarian café-cum-bakery, which serves delicious and healthful vegetarian food, fusing Japanese, Chinese, and American cuisines.

The cafe and bakery are on the site of her former design studio in which she turned out the dress designs that made her one of the world's top Chinese-American fashion designers. As befits such a gifted artisan, the interior is elegantly designed, and the walls are adorned with her hand-painted murals and sumi-e paintings. But why, we wondered, did she give up such an enviable career?

Nonplussed, we overcame our reticence and asked her why she would have forsaken her successful fashion-designing business to become a full-time baker, chef, and restaurant owner. She told us that as a devout Buddhist she felt a special calling, actuated by the first precept of *ahimsa,* to try to help enlighten the public by purveying healthful vegetarian food and providing them with instruction on how to prepare it. To that end, she offers free cooking classes every Sunday afternoon.

We started with a cup of carrot soup, which was a bit plain but bracing. Then we had the Sesame Vegi "Beef" on Rice, which was very tasty indeed. This was followed by Vegetarian Rice Noodles, and Vegi Beef Noodles—two dishes that had the savory goodness of home-cooked food. That same wholesome savoriness characterized all the dishes we tried–the Buckwheat noodles with three kinds of vegetables and five spices, and the Potato Salad featuring parti-colored potatoes-white, red, pink and purple—that were bursting with flavor.

For dessert, we particularly relished the walnut pie. And the organic coffee, which is made with Kangen water—[That is, water that has been alkalinized by a special machine that was invented by a Japanese doctor, Dr. Kangen.]--was superb coffee, In fact we can say, without hyperbole, it is the best we've ever tasted. (Must have been the Kangen water?)

Most of her pastries are vegan, but a few, unaccountably, are made with eggs [Eggs are not Buddhist!]. No other animal ingredients were used in their preparation; so we were somewhat baffled by their incongruous presence on the menu. Otherwise, the food is vegan.

Just inside the entrance there is large refrigerator case for those whose tastes run to exotic mock meats. It is crammed with such delicacies as Vegi Ribbon Fish, Vegi Eel, Vegi Beggar's Chicken and Vegi Black Pepper Steak. Bread. A Café', which is a pun on Brenda's name, is a must for those who love healthful vegetarian Chinese home-style cuisine. No gratuities are accepted.

BUDDHA BODAI [v] $

	42-96 Main Street
Full service	at Cherry Avenue
Chinese (kosher)	718-939-1188
$7.95-14.95 (all cards)	daily 11am-11pm
No alcohol.	

There is a wide array of dishes to choose from--Veg. Snail to Sweet and Sour Fish. Indeed, the range of ersatz is so exhaustive that it put us in mind of those Taoist temple kitchens in which chefs flaunt their ingenuity by creating ever more elaborate mock meat dishes. But we did not enjoy our dining experience here; mainly because the manager was brusque and discourteous and refused to entertain any questions as to which dishes were vegan and which were not.

DIMPLE INDIAN FAST FOOD [v] $

	35-68 73rd Street
Counter service	at 37th Avenue
Indian Vegetarian	718-458-8144

For description and hours, see the Manhattan listing under Midtown East.

DOSA DINER [v] **$**
Full service
South Indian
$4-5 (no cards)
No alcohol

35-66 73rd Street
at 37th Avenue
718-205-2218
11:30am-10pm

"Nothing could be finer than dosas from this diner" is a ditty that one might recite after eating the dosas here. We highly recommend the Vegetable Dosa and the Vegetables Uthappam. In Jackson Heights, the uthappams and the dosas are bigger, the fillings more generous, and the food spicier, but also more dairy-laden than in Manhattan. The saving grace is that the prices are much more reasonable out here than in the Big Dosa.

DOSA HUTT [v] **$**

Counter service
South Indian Vegetarian
$3.00-8.00 (no cards)
No alcohol

45-63 Bowne Street
(Flushing)
718-961-5897
daily 10am-9pm

This is India's answer to the Pizza Hut. Dosas, which are enormous crepes filled with spicy potato mixtures, do bear a resemblance to pizza, but I'll take a dosa over a pizza any time. The dosas here are tip-top, We especially relished the Masala Dosa. As with Dossa Diner, they're biigger and cheaper here than in the Big Dosa!

EXOTIC SUPERFOODS [v] **$** 👍

Counter service
Organic rawfoods
All Cards
No alcohol

185-02 Horace Harding Expwy
at 186th Street
718-353-4807
M-Sa 9am-10pm

Our visit to Exotic Superfoods (via the number 7 train from Grand Central to Main Street Flushing and the Q17 bus) was strenuous, but well worth the effort. Li, one of the four owners, a vivacious Chinese-American lady, made us a delicious raw salad, which contained mixed greens, dulse, grated carrots, goji berries, pine nuts, avocados, topped off with a hot and sour dressing. If there is a tastier salad in all of New York, we would like to know of it.

The owners who double as waiters and chefs and factota, are friendly, smiling and unfailingly courteous. They behave as if they really love what they are doing.

Matt, who is Li's husband, is the main rawfoods chef. He studied locally with raw master chefs Mary Trimble, Jeremy Safron, and David Jubb. But his creations bid fair to outstrip those of his masters. Our taste buds vibrated to the flavor notes of his raw Veggie Burger (almond cheese, red sauce and marinated sweet onions on a live organic flax cracker). We also deeply delighted in his raw Pizza. The crust is made of buckwheat, flaxseeds, Italian herbs, sun-dried tomatoes, garlic oil and Celtic sea salt. It is layered with almond cheese, spaghetti sauce, bell pepper, onions and sun-dried tomatoes.

For dessert, we inhaled Matt's Mamey Pie, which is close kin to that old Southern standby Sweet Potato Pie. Only this is the raw equivalent. Mamey is a tropical fruit in the Sapote family. Its reddish-orange pulp looks and tastes just like sweet potato. ·

Not to be missed are the smoothies. We had the house smoothie, which contains the following uplifting ingredients: organic apple juice, frozen plantain, acai, cacao nibs, coconut butter goji berries, mocha, spirulina and vanilla bean. After quaffing this, we were ready to levitate..

It is not hyperbole when we state that the fare at Exotic Superfoods is the best vegan rawfood to be had in all five boroughs, at a fraction of the prices charged by such posh rawfoods eateries in Manhattan. as Pure Food and Wine!

HAPPY BUDDHA [ve] $

Full service
Chinese
All major cards
No alcohol
www.happybuddha.com

135-37 37th Avenue
(Flushing)
718-358-0079
daily 11am-10pm

There are a myriad of tasty dishes on the menu that would make the Buddha and any other vegetarian very happy indeed. The Vegetarian Mock Duck was a personal favorite.

LINDA'S ORGANIC KITCHEN AND MARKET [ve]] $

Buffet./counter service
International, American
$3.00-6.00 (all cards)
No alcohol

81-22 Lefferts Boulevard
bet. Austin Street//83rd Avenue
718-847-2233
M-F 10am-7pm
Sa 10am-6pm; Su 11am-5:30pm

While you're shopping at Linda's Organic Market, in the tree-fringed streets of Kew Gardens, it's nice to know that you can grab a quick bite just a few steps away at Linda's Organic Kitchen. Like Integral Yoga, Linda's has a vegetarian deli and juice bar where you may indulge your appetite without compromising your karma. The vegan desserts are baked daily. Linda, who grew up in Hawaii, exudes good health, and has a sunny personality. She, herself, prepares all the yummy dishes--from casseroles to sandwiches, to fruit pies. If you're a salad lover, you're in luck. Linda prepares composed salads such as Quinoa Salad, Artichoke Salad, and Vegan Sushi.

VISIT
WOODSTOCK FARM ANIMAL SANCTUARY

Over 140 Rescued Farm Animals
2 Hours from NYC in Scenic Woodstock, NY
Open April - October (Volunteers Year-Round)
Direct Trailways Bus Service

MAHARAJAH QUALITY [v] $
SWEETS & SNACKS

Full service
International vegetarian
$400-12.00 (all cards)
No alcohol

73-10 37th Avenue
bet. 73rd/ 74th Streets
718-505-2680
daily 10am-10pm

As with Shamiana, this is Indian cuisine at its most caseous. The sweets and the dishes in the back are awash in milk, yogurt, cream, ghee, butter and cheese. You can pick your way through the menu to find vegan dishes, but is it really worth it?

ONENESS FOUNTAIN HEART [v] $$

Full service
International vegetarian
$400-12.00 (all cards)
No alcohol

157-19 72md Avenue
(Flushing)
718-591-3663
daily 11:30-9pm
W 11:00-9:00

Yet another restaurant that is operated by disciples of Sri Chimnoy. In addition to the -blue facades that all the restaurants share, they also have in common an uncommon devotion to high culinary standards and service. The dishes to try here are the Duck Surprise, which is made with vegetarian mock duck, and the Vegetarian Meatloaf. My personal favorite was Thai Heaven, which consists of spicy tofu skin in a delicate coconut sauce. It's worth taking a cab from Manhattan for this one.

SMILE OF THE BEYOND [v] $$

Counter service
International vegetarian
$4.00-6.00 (no cards)
No alcohol

86-14 Parsons Boulevard
(Jamaica)
718-739-7453
M-F 7am-4pm
Sa 7am-3pm

Not all restaurants in Queens are run by followers of Sri Chimnoy, it only seems that way. This astoundingly inexpensive luncheonette serves delicious veggie burgers, and generous salads that would cost the earth in a Manhattan eatery. All three Chimnoy places are worth the trek from Manhattan. At this place, so economical are the prices that the train fare will probably end up costing more than the meal!

THERESA'S VEGETARIAN CREATIONS [v] $

Buffet./counter service
International, American
All cards
No alcohol

21713 Jamaica Avenue
bet. 217th/ 218th Streets
718-464-7100
M-Th 9am-7:30pm
F 7am-5pm

A devout 7th-Day Adventist, Theresa seemed to bristle when we asked her if her food was "Ital." She grew up in the Virgin Islands and has arrived at her vegetarianism via the teachings of Sister Ellen White and Dr. John Harvey Kellogg. Nonetheless, her mostly vegan cuisine can stand comparison with the best Ital chefs in Harlem and Brooklyn. We especially savored the Sweet 'N' Sour Tofu, Vegetarian Soy Chunks, and the Chick-Pea Balls. Her repertoire of tasty vegan dishes is vast, and the menu changes daily. It's best to arrive early for lunch and early for dinner because her delectable dishes are snapped up quickly.

VEGGIE CASTLE [ve] $

Counter service
Caribbean
All cards
No alcohol

132-091 Liberty Avenue
near Van Wyck Expwy
718-641-8342
daily 10am-10pm

Last year Veggie Castle moved to Queens from its original location in Brooklyn, where it had struck a decided blow for veganism and animal rights by turning a White Castle fast food restaurant into a vegan Rasta restaurant. When Veggie Castle first opened, it was as though the farm animals had revolted and taken over the farm! The hostages had overpowered their captors!

Some enterprising vegetarian business folks had actually taken over a former burger joint and turned it into a vegetarian restaurant that serves the Veggie Castle Burger along with an array of delicious dishes that you won't find in your typical fast food place--such as Curried Soy Chicken, BRQ Soy Chunks With Pineapple, and ersatz Shepherd's Pie. We had a Spicy Black Bean Burger that was much the best veggie burger we'd ever tasted. We followed this with an order of Turmeric Bean Curd Duck that really showed off to advantage the culinary talent of Veggie Castle's Rasta *chefs de cuisine*. Instead of soda pop and shakes, Veggie Castle's juice bar serves a range of fresh fruit/vegetable juices and smoothies. Veggie Castle is giving fast food such a good name that, in the future, all burger joints may be dishing up Wheat Grass Juice and Veggie Burgers. It's cause for hope.

THE BRONX

H.I.M. |v| **$**
Counter service
Organic Caribbean
All Cards
No alcohol

754 Burke Avenue
Bronx
718-653-9627
daily 10am-9pm

The Bronx's first vegan restaurant is H.I.M. No, it's not a sexist cabal. H.I.M. is an acronym for His Imperial Highness, Hailie Selasie, the late emperor of Ethiopia who is regarded as the founding prophet of Rastafarianism. Rastafarians abstain from alcohol and all animal flesh. Pictures of Haile Selassie and other famous Rastafarians festoon the walls. Nazar, the Antiguan native who owns H.I.M., is a very religious guy who infuses his food with ethereal flavors. The menu changes every day, but the dishes we sampled were all pretty tasty. Among them were the Rasta standards: Barbecued Vegi Chicken, Kalaloo, Scrambled Tofu, Tofu Balls, Yam and Tofu Stew. For dessert, we had a slice of Almond Cake and a Mango Turnover. From the outside, H.I.M. looks a bit unkempt, and from the inside it also looks unkempt, but the food is good. Whether you're a HIM or a HER, if you're a connoisseur of pretty good vegan food, you should hasten to H.I.M.

VEGAN'S DELIGHT |v| **$$**
Counter service
Organic Caribbean
All Cards
No alcohol

3565 Boston Road
at Tiemann Avenue
718-653-4140
M-Sa 8am-6:30pm

Like Healthy Pleasure and Imhoteps, in Queens and Brooklyn, respectively, Vegan's Delight is a combination health-food store and restaurant. Is it worth the trip from Manhattan to eat here? That depends: If you're a connoisseur of Ital food as we are, then the trip is certainly warranted. However, there are places in Manhattan and Brooklyn that do the Ital thing just as well if not better. For instance: The Uptown Juice Bar and Veggie Castle--to list but two. We savored the Curried Bean Curd, the Ital Stew, and the Eggplant Melange, and commend it to you.

WOODSTOCK

GARDEN CAFE [v] $$

Full service
Global Organic
All cards
Organic wines & beers

6 Old Forge Road
(on the Village Green)
845-679-3600
W-M 11:30am-9pm

One of our favorite New York escapes is to spend the weekend in Woodstock. It is still redolent of the arts colony that it used to be in the early part of the last century, and of the hippie era of the sixties. Now we can augment the pleasure of our weekend getaways by dining at the Garden Café. It was opened two years ago by chef Pam Brown. She earned her stripes as a chef at the Great Sage Café in Baltimore, where she trained under master macrobiotic chef Hiroshi Hyashi.

In keeping with the macrobiotic spirit of her mentor, she advocates eating locally grown produce. All the ingredients in her dishes are as pure, natural, and organic as possible.

In addition to her regular lunch and dinner menus, daily specials include a Garden Bowl, consisting of greens, whole grains, vegetables, beans, tofu, tempeh, or seitan. We started with the Moroccan Carrot Salad with Pistachio and Dates. *Extraordinare!*

Then we tucked into an international array of dishes that included Indian Vegetable and Chickpea Enchiladas, served with a Bombay Sauce, and a Curried Apple-Coconut Salad on the side. *Sensationel!* We also had the Southwest Black Bean and Roasted Sweet Potato Burger with Guacamole Salsa and a wedge of Vegan Cheddar. *Magnifique!* After downing these, our faces beamed with satisfaction.

We had to bolt in order to be on time for a concert at the Maverick; so we skipped the Warm Chocolate Brownie with Hot Fudge Sauce, served with Vegan Whipped Cream, and the Raw Agave Pistachio Gelato. But we will be returning tomorrow night, [after we visit the Woodstock Farm Animal Sanctuary, and the Catskill Animal Sanctuary], to sit in reposeful ease under the poplar trees and gaze at the town square "thinking green thoughts in a green shade."

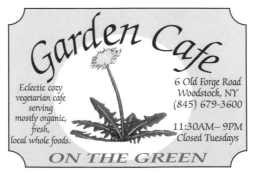

Garden Cafe

Eclectic cozy
vegetarian cafe
serving
mostly organic,
fresh,
local whole foods.

6 Old Forge Road
Woodstock, NY
(845) 679-3600

11:30AM– 9PM
Closed Tuesdays

ON THE GREEN

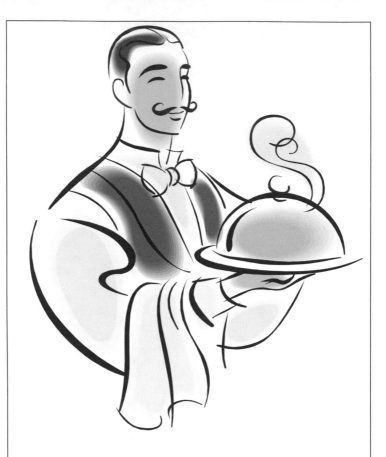

"The discovery of a new vegan restaurant dish does more for the well-being of the human race than the discovery of a new star."

...Jean Brillat Savarin (1756-1825)
[revised with apologies]

CYBERSPACE

VEGGIE BROTHERS.COM [v] $$C

Shipped frozen to your door
Global vegan, organic
All Cards
No alcohol

www.veggiebrothers.com
in cyberspacce
877-VEGAN-55
daily 24hours

Now you have no excuse for not sticking to a vegan diet even in the remotest hinterlands. Veggie Brothers, the first online gourmet vegan restaurant, employs chef Mark Rasmussen to whip up the most sumptuous vegan meals this side of Vegan Paradise. Just place your order 24 hours in advance and wait for your meal to arrive. Choose from a delicious array of over thirty healthful chef-crafted options. Each selection is available in single, family, or catering portion sizes. We tried the vegan Ole El Paso Stew and the Tempeh Parmeghana, and fancied that we were in one of the world's great vegan restaurants--Candle 79, Franchia, Caravan of Dreams, in Manhattan, or Vegethus in Sao Paulo. We also savored their Manchurian Pepper Steak (with a side of brown rice). It was on sale as a daily special. Made from seitan, it was so artfully prepared that we had the illusion of dining at Zen Palate Only the glare of the flashing neon light reminded us that we were stopping for two nights at a Red Roof Inn, a thousand miles from the nearest vegan restaurant.

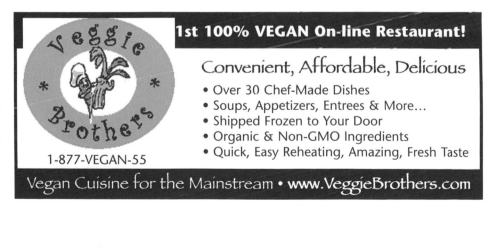

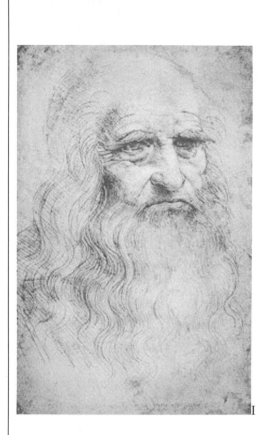

I have from an early age abjured the use of meat, and the time will come when men such as I will look upon the murder of animals as they now look upon the murder of men.

LEONARDO DA VINCI, 1452-1519
Artist, scientist, inventor, engineer, architect
"Renaissance Man"

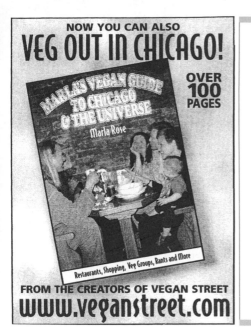
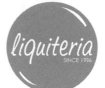
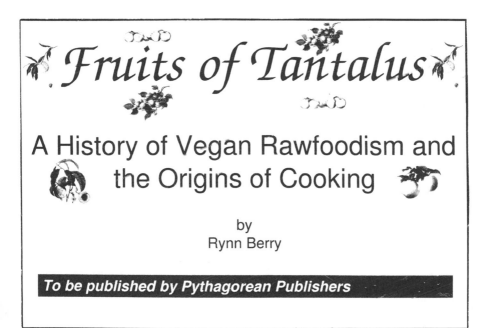

Fruits of Tantalus

A History of Vegan Rawfoodism and the Origins of Cooking

by
Rynn Berry

To be published by Pythagorean Publishers

TOP TEN JUICE BARS

U
O

Although they don't yet outnumber the alcohol bars, or the coffee bars, juice bars are starting to crop up all over town. Unhappily, many of them--like Gray's Papaya--serve meat along with their smoothies and juices. [Recently, we had to drop Juice Generation for serving Chicken Sandwiches.] So we picked places that serve only vegan dishes to go with their drinks. Not so long ago, New Yorkers used to start the day with a shot of bourbon or a mug of java; now, as like as not, they'll get their hearts started with a shot of "green plasma"--wheat grass juice, brimming with enzymes, anti-oxidants, chlorophyll, and phytonutrients.

DOUG GREEN'S LIQUITERIA [v]
170 2nd Avenue
bet. 11th and 12th Streets
daily 8am-10:30pm

The standard by which all others are measured. The best smoothies in the universe! This is the only juice bar in the city that uses 100% organic, fresh fruits and juices.

Doug's criteria for hygiene and service are exacting. Working surfaces and equipment are constantly being scrubbed with an unsleeping vigilance. Well-mannered, eager-to-please, and efficient, his staff clearly love their work as most have been in Doug's employ for six years!

His is the only juice bar in the city that uses a Norwalk hydraulic press. (Up to five times more of the enzymes, minerals and vitamins are expressed in the juices by this method than by any other.) For a bracing sandwich, try Doug's Tempeh Bacon Lettuce and Tomato. For a Smoothie, try the Papaya Paradise (papaya peaches, banana, apple cider, vanilla soy milk, shredded coconut) They're a ticket to esophageal paradise.

EXOTIC SUPERFOODS [v]
185-02 Horace Harding Expwy
at 186th Street
M-Sa 9am-10pm

Not to be missed are the fruit smoothies. We had the house smoothie, which contains the following uplifting ingredients: organic apple juice, frozen plantain, acai, cacao nibs, coconut butter goji berries, mocha, spirulina and vanilla bean. After quaffing this, we were ready to levitate..

JUBB'S LONGEVITY [v]
508 East 12th Street
bet. Avenues A/ B
daily 10am-9pm

Dr. David Jubb is as much an alchemist with juices and smoothies as he is with food. Try his incomparable Amazon fruit smoothies such as the Acai, or the Passion Fruit. Or have his Mixed Berry Smoothie. Have a raw vegan Burger Deluxe for David's unfired vegan version of the all American combo of Burger 'n' Shake.

RAW SOUL[v]

348 West 145th Street
bet. St. Nicholas/ Edgecomb
daily 9:am-9pm

This rawfood delicatessen-cum-juice bar offers a range of juices and juice combinations along with salads and some tasty raw fruit pies. Try Island Spice (pineapple, papaya, mango, ginger root), or Berry, Berry, Berry Good (strawberry, blueberry and raspberry).It and some of the daily specials like the Personal Pizza, are indeed Berry, Berry, Berry good!

.

PERELANDRA [v] $C

175 Remsen Street
bet. Court/ Clinton
718-855-6068
M-F 8:30-8:30
Sa 9:30-8:30:
Su 11-7

For the post prandial beverage, we sipped their Avocado Smoothie. Which contains Coconut Juice, Avocado, Agave Nectar, and Fresh Lime Juice. We specifically requested that they make it with Agave nectar as they ordinarily make it with honey.

JUS [v]

16th Street
at Union Square West,
daily 8am-8pm

Joao, the Brazilian man who runs this stand, concocts delicious smoothies and fruit tonics. His best-selling fruit tonic is an apple-cantaloupe, pineapple combo; and his best-selling smoothie is mango, strawberry and pineapple. It's our favorite as well.

GREENER PASTURES [ve]

Union Square Greenmarket
16th St. / Union Square West
M,W, F, Sa 8am-7pm

On Mondays, Wednesdays, Fridays and Saturdays of every week, Stewart, the proprietor, serves up wheat grass juice and effervescent good humor to the patrons who mob his stand. They swear he has the sweetest grass in the city. A one ounce shot is $2.00 a double shot is $3.50. Stewart also sells flats of Wheat Grass as well as succulent salad greens.

UPTOWN JUICE BAR [ve]

54 West 125th Street
daily 8am-10pm

They offer a wide array of juices and juice combinations that are designed to cure everything from asthma to impotence. The fruit smoothes are delicious, and the Caribbean style vegan food is first rate.

FOOD SHOPPING

I't's possible to eat cheaply in New York. It's also possible to spend your life savings on a single meal (though much easier for meat-eaters than for vegans!). This applies to restaurants as well as to shops, which range from the most luxurious importers to inexpensive, dependable local farm products. Below are some notable places that won't break your budget; for obvious reasons, this is not a comprehensive list. Individual addresses are listed on the following page.

SUPERMARKETS

these, and it The largest stores carry health food items, soy milk, and the like, but their prices are not usually any lower than large health food shops for these goods. The New York chains, listed in roughly ascending order of price (quality is quite similar): Associated, Sloan's, Gristede's, Met Food, D'Agostino, Food Emporium, WholeFoods.

PRODUCE

There are greenmarkets, also called farmer's markets, on certain days in public squares, where producers drive truckloads of fresh and often organic fruits and vegetables into the city from their farms in upstate New York, Pennsylvania, and New Jersey. The prices and quality can't be beat, and there's a festive atmosphere to these events. Of course, you'll find only what's in season, so there are slim pickings during the cold winter months. Union Square is the largest of boasts a vegan bakery stall called Body & Soul with great treats both sweet and savory.

The next choice for organic produce is shopping at a large health food store like Wholesome Market, Integral Yoga or Commodities. Prices are a bit higher, but the quality is excellent.

For non-organic produce, the Asian shops along Canal Street in Chinatown and on First Avenue around 7th Street in the East Village have the lowest prices. Otherwise, supermarkets and the 24-hour groceries that line many New York streets are fairly reliable.

BULK GOODS, SPICES, ETC.

The larger health food shops all have a section where you can buy grains, beans, nuts, dried fruit, flour and snacks in bulk, most of it organic. For non-organic bulk goods and wonderful spices at low prices, try the Indian shops around Lexington and 28th Street or First Avenue and 6th Street.

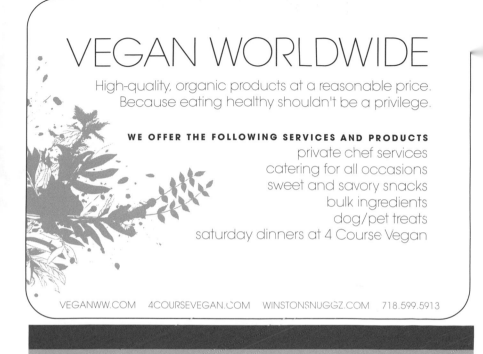

FAVORITE SHOPS

HARLEM

FAIRWAY FRUITS & VEGETABLES
Huge produce and natural food store.

2328 Twelfth Avenue
at West 132nd Street

7 GRAINS HEALTH FOODS
Health food shop.

2259 Seventh Avenue
at 133rd Street

UPPER WEST SIDE

CREATIVE
Health food shop.

2805 Broadway
bet. 108th/109th Streets

GARY NULL'S UPTOWN WHOLEFOODS
2307 Broadway
at West 89th Street
Health food grocery with bustling juice bar and kosher vegetarian salad bar.

HEALTH NUTS
Health food shop with juice bar.

2611 Broadway
at West 99th Street

OLIVIERS & CO
Olive oil shop.'

198 Columbus Avenue
at 69th Street

WHOLEFOODS MARKET
Organic supermarket.

10 Columbus Circle
at 60th Street

UPPER EAST SIDE

HEALTH NUTS

1208 Second Avenue

Health food shop with juice bar.

bet. 63rd/64th Streets

MATTER OF HEALTH
Health food shop with juice bar.

1478 First Avenue
at 77th Street

NATURAL FRONTIER
Organic grocery with emphasis on vegetarian and vegan.

1424 Third Avenue
at 81st Street

MIDTOWN WEST

HEALTHY CHELSEA
Health food shop with juice bar.

248 West 23rd Street
bet. Seventh/Eighth Avenues

NICE N' NATURAL
Health food shop with juice bar.

673 Ninth Avenue
bet. 46th / 47th Streets

ORGANIC MARKET
Health food shop.

229 Seventh Avenue
bet. 23rd/24th Streets

SIVANANDA YOGA VEDANTA CENTER
Exercise, breathing, relaxation, diet, and mediation

243 West 24th Street
bet. 7th/8th Avenues

WESTERLY NATURAL MARKET
Well stocked organic grocery.

911 Eighth Avenue
at 54th Street

WHOLEFOODS MARKET
Organic supermarket.

250 Seventh Avenue
at 24th Street

MIDTOWN EAST

BETH'S FARM KITCHEN
Jams, jellies and pickled vegetables F, Sa year-round.

Union Square Greenmarket
bet. 17th St / Union Sq.West

BODY & SOUL
All-vegan baked goods stand.M F year-round.

Union Square Greenmarket
bet. 17th St / Union Sq.West

FANTASY FRUIT FARM
Blueberries, strawberries, raspberries, seedless grapes
Saturdays, June-Nov.

Union Square Greenmarket
bet. 17th St. / Union Sq. West

...S OF INDIA
...er Indian grocery.

121 Lexington Avenue
bet. 29th/30th Streets

...ALTH NUTS
...ell-provisioned health food store.

835 2nd Avenue
bet. 44th/ 45th Streets

KALUSTYAN

123 Lexington Avenue
bet. 28th / 29th Streets

Well-stocked Indian Grocery. They feature bulk items such as raw pistachio nuts and sun-dried strawberries.

KEITH'S FARM
Heirloom herbs, garlics and greens, We Sa, Ju -Nov.

Union Square Greenmarket
bet. 17th St. / Union Sq. West

LOCUST GROVE FRUIT FARM
A cornucopia of delicious fruit, W, Sa year-round.

Union Square Greenmarket
bet. 17th St. / Union Sq. West

OLIVIERS & CO
Olive oil merchants

Grand Central Terminal
near Track 17

This store specializes in premium olive oils from all the Mediterranean countries plus Uruguay. They also sell a highly addictive sun-dried tomato powder for sprinkling on salads and suchlike vegan fare.

PHILLIPS FARMS
:

Union Square Greenmarket
bet. 17th/ Union Sq. West

Peaches, Raspberries, Blueberries and Blackberries. March-December, M, Sa 8am-6pm.

RICK'S PICKS

Union Square Greenmarket
bet. 17th/ Union Sq. West

Rick, an Andover and Yale alum, quit his job as PBS producer to become a picklemeister. Favorite pickle is Wasabean (green beans and wasabi). Wednesdays sunrise to sunset, year round.

TRADER JOE'S

142 East 14th Street
at Union Sq. East

An offbeat supermarket, Joe's is famous for its unusual and inexpensive products, like wild blueberry juice, dark chocolate-covered espresso beans, and, our favorite, chili-spiced dried mango slices.

WINDFALL FARM
Wide range of organic greens, We, Sa year round

Union Square Greenmarket
bet. 17th St. / Union Sq. West

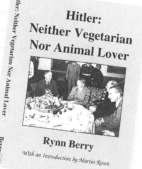

:EGRAL YOGA NATURAL FOODS 229 West 13th Street
:alth food shop bet. Seventh/Eighth Avenues
Jood quality and price on organics and bulk goods, plus hot and cold buffet. Some raw food
dishes. Very popular.

LIFETHYME 410 Sixth Avenue
at Eighth Street
One-stop shopping for large selection of exclusively organic produce, bulk goods, vitamins,
herbal nostrums, and cruelty-free cosmetics. Amazing salad bar and delicious vegetarian food to
go. Their vegan bakery turns out scrumptious pastries and prides itself on not using milk eggs or
cheese in any of their cakes cookies or pies. They have a spiffy juice bar, and a good selection
of books on nutrition and healing. Recently, they've added a living foods section with delicious
raw pies, cakes and entrees.

NY ARTIFICIAL 223 West 10th Street

NYA BLUE 13 8th Avenue
At West 12th Street
NYA GREEN 13 8th Avenue
At West 12th Street
Handbags, jewelry, accessories,, shoes, apparel, and makeup.
www. nyartificial.com • 646-340-0442 • 646-340-0813

OLIVIERS & CO, 249 Bleecker Street
Olive oil merchants. bet. 7th / 6th Avenues

ORGANIC MARKET 250 Mercer Street
Large health food shop with bulk section and juice bar. bet. 3rd/4th Streets

STELLA McCARTNEY 429 West 14th Street
bet. 9th/ 10th Avenues
The scion of Sir Paul sells vegan shoes and cruelty-free clothing of her own design.

EAST VILLAGE

ANGELICA'S 147 First Avenue
Herbs at 9th Street
One of the largest selections of herbs, both culinary and medicinal, expensive organic produce.

COMMODITIES EAST 165 First Avenue

at 10th Street
Health food shop with good quality and prices on organic produce and bulk goods.

4TH STREET FOOD COOP   58 East Fourth Street
                                         bet. Bowery and Second
All produce from leafy greens to tubers is organic, and the granola, grains, nuts and other bulk
times are mostly so. Non-members are welcome.

HIGH VIBE HEALTH & HEALING   138 East Third Street (rear)
                                         bet. 1st / A Avenues
A raw food superstore since '93 created by Bob Dagger, who has collected and created some of
the largest selections of rawfood snacks, food, supplements, super foods, appliances, potions,
books, beauty care, along with his nutritional counseling and classes; your one stop for
everything you need for better health. A must visit also on line for great free recipes and free
information: highvibe.com.

INDIA SPICE HOUSE   99 First Avenue
Indian grocery, 24 hours   at 6th Street
Smaller than the Lexington stores, and the foodstuffs don't move so quickly, but still good—
especially if you need some fenugreek or asafoetida in the middle of the night. 400 kinds of beer.

JUBB'S LONGEVITY   508 E. 12th Street
                                         bet. Avenues A / B
Living foods patisserie, life food preparation classes, and a range of super foods and cosmetic
products that purport to promote longevity.Try Jubb's Body Ice; and Essential Oils.

JIVAMUKTI YOGA CENTER   841 Broadway
                                         bet. 13th/ 14th Streets
Yoga Center and emporium that sells yoga paraphernalia, eco-friendly clothing, books. It also
features a new vegan cafe -cum-juice bar called JivamukTea, Try the Raw Lasagna, the Creator
BLT, and chef Matthew Kenney's delicious raw desserts.

LIVE LIVE   261 East 10th Street
                                         bet. 1st Avenue / Avenue A
Raw foods boutique, featuring, a wide selection of books, super foods, snacks, potions,
energizers and rejuvenatives. Also on sale are dehydrators, juicers and other accouterments of
the raw food lifestyle.

SUSTAINABLE NYC   147 Avenue A
                                         bet. 9th/ 10th Streets
Local, organic, re-cycled, fair-trade, re-purposed, biodegradable, products and gifts.

...EFOODS UNION SQUARE
...supermarket.

40 East 14th Street
at Broadway

SOHO

BABY CAKES
Vegan baked goods.

240 Broome Street
bet. Orchard/ Ludlow Streets

EKOVARUHUSET
Organic, fair trade clothing

123 Ludlow Street

EARTH MATTERS
Organic market with salad bar

177 Ludlow Street
bet. Stanton/ Houston

GUSS'S LOWER EAST SIDE PICKLES

85-87 Orchard Street
bet. Broome/ Grand

Pickled tomatoes, artichoke hearts as well the old standbys. This shop and its owner starred in the motion picture Crossing Delancey Street.

MAY WAH HEALTHY VEG. FOOD

213 Hester Street
bet. Centre / Baxter

Chinese Vegetarian grocery store. Well-stocked with mock meats such as mock shrimp, mock duck, mock squid, etc.

MOO SHOES

78 Orchard Street
bet. Stanton/ Rivington

The best selection of cruelty-free shoes and accessories in the country.

ORGANIC AVENUE

01 Stanton Street
bet. Orchard/ Ludlow

Hemp and organic clothing, organic lifestyle products, fresh, raw and organic produce collective.

WHOLEFOODS MARKET
Organic supermarket.

95 East Houston Street
at Bowery

BELOW CANAL STREET

BELL BATES
Large Health Food Grocery Store

97 Reade Street
bet. W.Bway / Church

Rynn Berry

Food for the Gods

Vegetarianism & the World's Religions

384 pages 0-9626169-2-3 $19.95 paperback

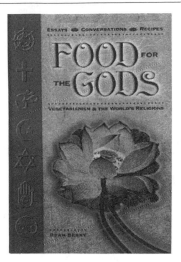

"*Food for the Gods* is eloquently philosophical; it is eavesdropping on the erudite."—**Dr. Kristin Aronson**, Professor of Philosophy, Western Connecticut University

"Rynn Berry has created a memorable feast for mind, body, and soul. *Food for the Gods* makes a tasty and terrific gift for the cook who has everything, including a lively curiosity and an adventurous culinary spirit."—**Lorna Sass**, author of *Lorna Sass' Complete Vegetarian Kitchen*

"The aptly named Rynn Berry has become the official vegan ambassador. His books treat vegetarianism not merely as a cult but as a culture. For Berry, the act of eating is not just a matter of sustenance, it's also a novel and even a spiritual act. His latest, *Food for the Gods*, is a fascinating investigation into the world's great religions. Berry provides illuminating essays on vegetarianism in Jainism, Hinduism, Buddhism, Sufism, and other non-Western religions, as well as Christianity and Judaism. He interviews religious thinkers who are also vegetarians, and he supplies recipes for dishes that have come from these different cultures. The result is a banquet for the taste buds of the mind."—**Jack Kroll**, Senior Editor *Newsweek*

Rynn Berry is the historical advisor to the North American Vegetarian Society and the author of *The New Vegetarians* and *Famous Vegetarians and Their Favorite Recipes*, a biographical history of vegetarianism that ranges from Pythagoras and the Buddha through to Isaac Bashevis Singer and the Beatles. He lives in Brooklyn.

<u>Also by Rynn Berry</u>:
Famous Vegetarians and Their Favorite Recipes: Lives and Lore from the Buddha to the Beatles
The New Vegetarians

Berry, *Food for the Gods* 0-9626169-2-3 $19.95 paperback

I enclose a check for $:___ _____

Tel #:___ _____

Shipping: $3.00 for one book, $1.00 for each additional book

TOTAL ENCLOSED	$

Name:_____

Address: _____

City;_____State/Zip;_____

Send to:
Pythagorean Publishers
P.O. Box 8174, JAF Station, New York, NY 10116
Tel./Fax: 718-622-8002

MMODITIES NATURAL FOODS MARKET
st health food shop with good bulk prices.

117 Hudson Street
at North Moore Street

WHOLEFOODS MARKET
Organic supermarket

270 Greenwich Street

BROOKLYN

BACK TO THE LAND

142 Seventh Avenue
bet. Carroll Street/Garfield Place

Organically grown produce as well as grains, nuts and dried fruits are on offer. A wide range of books, magazines and tapes are for sale. There is a section for homeopathic remedies. And a well-stocked macro-biotic section.

DOWNTOWN NATURAL MARKET
Organic produce, Juice and Salad bars.

51 Willoughby Street
off Jay Street

FAIRWAY
The Manhattan food bazaar has come to Brooklyn.

480-500 Van Brunt Street
Red Hook

FORCES OF NATURE

1688 Sheepshead Bay Road

Organic Groceries, homeopathic remedies, books and music.

FLATBUSH FOOD COOP

1318 Corydon Road
bet.Rugby and Argyle Rds.

Fresh organic produce. Earth-friendly household products. Open to non-members

GOVINDA ORGANIC MARKET

387 Atlantic Avenue
bet. Hoyt/ Bond Streets

Orlando, the manager, who converted Westerly's from pharmacy to health food store, now has his own well-stocked health food market.

LIVING WELL NATURAL FOODS
Health food shop.

382 Seventh Avenue
at 12th Street

PARK SLOPE FOOD COOP
Members only organic market
Members pay 20% above cost. Closed to Non-members.

782 Union Street
bet. 6th & 7th Avenues

PERELANDRA NATURAL FOOD CENTER 175 Ramsen Street
at Court Street
Largest health food store in Brooklyn. Excellent juice bar and book section.

THE GARDEN 921 Manhattan Avenue
Well-stocked health food shop. at Kent Street (Willaimsburg)

QUEENS

BREAD. A BAKERY & CAFÉ 41-46 College Point Road
Bakery, café, and healthfood store bet. 41 Road/ Sanford

EXOTIC SUPERFOODS 185-02 Horce Harding Expwy
(Fresh Meadows)
GNOSIS CHOCOLATE (raw vegan chocolate) 40-03 27th Street
Long Island City
[Available at Westerly, High Vibe, Live Live, Jivamukti Yoga, & WholeFoods]

LINDA'S NATURAL MARKET 81-22 Lefferts Boulevard
Organic produce, vegetarian deli and juice bar. (Kew Gardens)

NEIL'S NATURAL MARKET 46-10 Hollis Court Avneue
(Flushing)
Organic produce, vitamins, rawfooods, herbs, homeopathy, cruelty-free body care products, and bulk items.

QUEENS HEALTH EMPORIUM 159-01 Horace Harding Expy.
Macrobiotic products, organic produce, juice bar. (Flushing Meadows).

THE BRONX

GOOD 'N' NATURAL 2173 White Plains Road
Exceptionally well stocked Health Food Store (bet. Pelham Pkwy/Lydig Ave)

One other place worth knowing about: Bruno Ravioli sells fresh and frozen pasta and offers a few amazing varieties of vegan ravioli to take home, like Shiitake Mushroom, Pumpkin, and Florentine (spinach and carrots). There are three stores: 235 East 22nd Street, 2204 Broadway, 1093 Lexington Avenue, and 249 Eighth Avenue.

RAW FOOD RESOURCES

✹

New York has not only the greatest wealth of vegan and vegetarian restaurants in the world, it also has the greatest wealth of rawfood resources. If you count Jubb's Longevity, and Caravan of Dreams, Bonobos, Liquiteria, and Jills, New York now boasts eleven raw food restaurants, and a growing number of raw food boutiques like High Vibe and Live Live, where the aspiring rawfooder may obtain nutritional guidance, instruction on raw food preparation, raw food snacks and useful gadgets like Food Processors, Saladacos (spiralizers). dehydrators, et al.

Restaurants

Bonobos Full raw menu	18 East 23rd Street bet. Park Avenue/Broadway
Caravan of Dreams Partial raw menu	405 East 6th Street bet. First Avenue / Avenue A
Exotic Superfoods 718-353-4807	185-02 Horace Harding Expwy (Fresh Meadows)
Jill's Hafl raw, half "kindly cooked"	23 Court Street bet. Warren/ Baltic Streets
Jubb's Longevity Full raw menu	508 East 12th Street bet. Avenues A/B
Doug Green's Liquiteria Best liquid raw food in town	170 2nd Avenue bet. 11th/12th
Pure Food and Wine The ne plus ultra of raw food restaurants	54 Irving Place bet. 17th/ 18th Streets
Pure Juice and Take Away The take-out editon of Pure Food and Wine	125 1/2 East 17th Street bet. 3rd Avenue / Irving Place
Quintessence Full raw menu	263 East 10th Street bet 1st Avenue / Avenue A

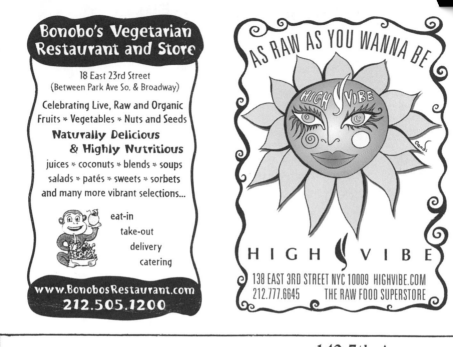
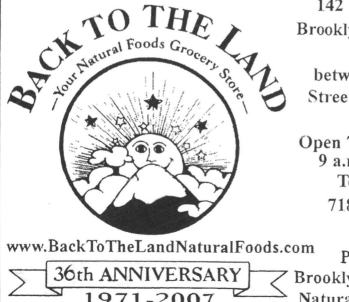

Soul
menu with juices and smoothies

348 West 145th Street
bet. St. Nicholas/ Edgecombe Avenues

.aw Star
Full raw menu with juices and smoothies

687 Washington Avenue
at Prsspect Place

Westerly Raw Food Bar
Raw food deli in NW corner of the store

911 Eighth Avenue
at 54th Street

Raw Boutiques

Raw boutiques hold lectures, food prep classes; and sell super foods, raw snacks, books, gadgets, cosmetics, and other adjuncts of the vegan rawfood lifestyle.

BONOBOS REAL FOOD STORE
212-505-1200

18 East 23rd Street
bet. Park Avenue/ Broadway

EXOTIC SUPERFOODS
718-353-4807

185-02 Horce Harding Expwy
(Fresh Meadows)

HIGH VIBE
212-777-6645

138 East 3rd Street
bet. First / A Avenues

JUBB'S LONGEVITY
212-353-5000

508 East 12th Street
bet. Avenues A/ B

LIVE LIVE
212-505-5504

261 East 10th Street
bet. 1st Avenue /Avenue A

ORGANIC AVENUE
212-334-4593

101 Stanton Street
bet. Orchard/ Ludlow

Rawfood Support Groups

NATURAL HYGIENE
212-956-2031

Mondays 7pm-9pm
416 West 46th Street

ACCENT ON WELLNESS
212 760-5953

Wednesdays 8pm-10pm
528 East 5th Street

Raw Vegan Chocolate

GNOSIS CHOCOLATE   Available at Westerly, High Vibe,
Live Live, Jivamukti Yoga, et al.

Raw Potlucks

MANHATTAN POTLUCK   First Saturday, Dharma Yoga Center
212-254-9453   297 Third Avenue

HALLELUJAH ACRES POTLUCK Last Sunday 484 West 43rs Street
212-594-0718   Apt. 34k (Rev. Lawrence Rush)

Hands On Raw Food Preparation Classes

JUBB'S LONGEVITY   212-353-5000

LIVE LIVE   212-505-5504

ORGANIC AVENUE   212-334-4593

QUINTESSENCE   212 501-9700

RAW SOUL   212-491-5859

RAW STAR   718-975-0304

Raw Foods on the Internet

HIGH VIBE   www. highvibe. com

NATURE'S FIRST LAW   www. rawfood.com

LIVING FOODS INSTITUTE   www.livingfoodsinstitute.com

HALLELUJAH ACRES   www. hacres.com

FRESH NETWORK   www. fresh-network.com

RAW NUTRTIONAL COUNSELING, www. doctorgraham.cc

...n Wigmore Natural Health Institute, PO Box 429, Rincon, PR 00677; (787) 868-6307
..he Annapurna Inn & Spa, 538 Adams, Port Townsend, WA 98368; (800) 868-ANNA.
Aris La Tham's SunJoy Natural Life Retreat, Coyaba Springs, River Gardens & Falls, Shaw
Park Ridge Estate, Ocho Rios, Jamaica (876) 441-0124, Sunfirefood@hotmail.com.
Vegan Living Foods Health Spa-Hippocrates Health Institute, 1441 Palmdale Court
West Palm Breach, FL 33411; (407) 471-8876
Vegan Health Spa-The Regency Health Spa, 2000 South Ocean Avenue, Hallandale,
FL 33009, (800) 454-0003
Water Fasting Center: True North, 4310 Lichau Road, Penngrove, CA 94951; (707) 792-2325
Living Foods Institute, 1530 Dekalb Avenue, Atlanta, GA 30307 • 800-844-9876

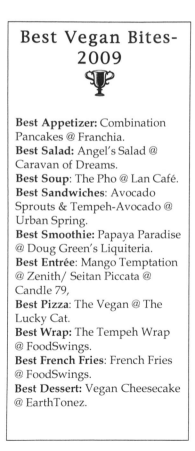

Best Vegan Bites- 2009

Best Appetizer: Combination
Pancakes @ Franchia.
Best Salad: Angel's Salad @
Caravan of Dreams.
Best Soup: The Pho @ Lan Café.
Best Sandwiches: Avocado
Sprouts & Tempeh-Avocado @
Urban Spring.
Best Smoothie: Papaya Paradise
@ Doug Green's Liquiteria.
Best Entrée: Mango Temptation
@ Zenith/ Seitan Piccata @
Candle 79,
Best Pizza: The Vegan @ The
Lucky Cat.
Best Wrap: The Tempeh Wrap
@ FoodSwings.
Best French Fries: French Fries
@ FoodSwings.
Best Dessert: Vegan Cheesecake
@ EarthTonez.

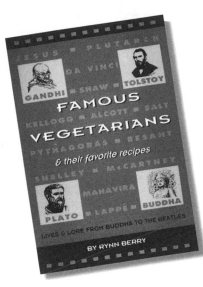

FAVORITE BOOKSTORES

New York is the national capital of the publishing world, and is full of bookstores of all types—large chains carrying bestsellers, small dusty used bookshops, specialized technical or foreign-language stores. Here are some of our hangouts.

ALABASTER BOOKS............................ 122 Fourth Avenue
Tel. 212- 982-3550   at 12th
BOOKCOURT................................... 363 Court Street
Tel. 718-875-3677   bet. Pacific/Dean
BLUESTOCKINGS............................... 172 Allen St.
Tel. 212-777-6028   bet. Stanton/Rivington Streets
COLISEUM BOOKS............................ .... 11 West 42nd Street
Tel. 212-840-7955   at Fifth Avenue
CRAWFORD-DOYLE............................ 1082 Madiosn Avenue
Tel. 212-288-6300   at 82nd Street
EAST WEST BOOKS............................. 78 Fifth Avenue
Tel. 212-243-5994   at 13th Street
GOTHAM...................................... 16 West 46th Street
Tel. 212-719-4448   bet. Fifth/Sixth Avenues
GRYPHON...................................... 233 West 72md Street
Tel. 212-874-1588   at Broadway
KITCHEN ARTS & LETTERS........................... 1435 Lexington
Tel. 212- 876-5550   at 94th Street
LABYRINTH BOOKS............................... 536 West 112th Street
Tel. 212-865-1588   bet. Broadway/Amsterdam Avenue
MERCER STREET BOOKS........................ 206 Mercer Street
Tel. 212-505-8615   at Bleecker
OPEN CENTER BOOKSTORE........................... 83 Spring Street
Tel. 212-219-2527 ext. 108   at Broadway
QUEST BOOKSHOP.............................. 240 East 53rd Street
Tel. 212- 758-5521   bet. Second/Third Avenues
SHAKESPEARE & CO............................ 716 Broadway
Tel. 212-529-1330   at Waverly Place
ST. MARK'S BOOKSHOP........................... 31 Third Avenue
Tel. 212-260-0443   at 9th Street
STRAND...................................... 828 Broadway
Tel. 212-473-1452   at 12th Street
THREE LIVES & CO............................ 154 West 10th Street
Tel. 212- 741-2069   at Waverly Place
USED BOOK CAFE............................... 120 Crosby Street
Tel. 212-334-3324   at Houston Street

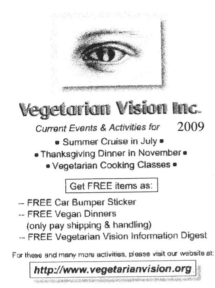
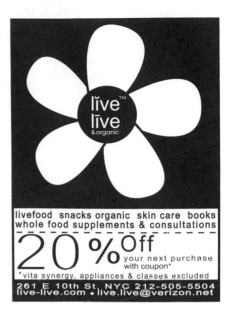
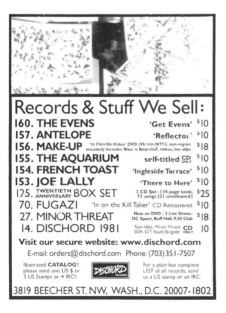

GLOSSARY

Baba ganoush	Middle Eastern spread made of eggplant, tahini, chick peas, lemon & garlic.
Bagel	The classic New York bread. Chewy and sprinkled with onion, garlic, or seeds, and shaped like a donut. Eat one and you won't be hungry for hours. Usually vegan; ask about eggs and egg glaze.
Casein	A milk protein that accounts for cheese's ability to melt smoothly. Alas, it is added to nearly all soy cheese, making it unacceptable for vegans.
Chips	To an American, chips are crisps and fries are chips. Get it?
Dim Sum	Asian buffet: a selection of lots of different dumplings, savory cakes and the like.
Eggplant	Aubergine.
Falafel	The vegetarian meatball: a Middle Eastern deep-fried patty of ground chick peas, garlic, and parsley.
Gluten	Chewy bland dough made from wheat flour which absorbs the flavors of the dish or sauce it's cooked in, like tofu. Common meat substitute.
Hummus	Middle Eastern spread made of ground chick peas, tahini, garlic, lemon and olive oil.
Knish	A savory pastry in which a simple thin dough is wrapped around a filling of potato, buckwheat, rice, etc. Usually vegan, but it pays to ask about cheese or butter, and whether the dough is made with egg.
Kosher	Strict dietary guidelines followed by some Jews; they include a prohibition on mixing meat with milk in the same meal or the same kitchen. That means a kosher "dairy" restaurant will have no meat, with lots of options for ovo-lacto vegetarians but nothing for vegans, while a kosher restaurant that serves meat will have no dairy. Likewise, if a processed food is labeled "kosher," it won't contain both animal gelatin and milk powder, for instance.
Macrobiotic	A way of eating from Eastern traditions that seeks to bring foods into balance. Macro restaurants usually serve fish and sometimes eggs, but no dairy; they always have plenty for vegans.

Pico de Gallo	Mexican salsa made from raw onions, tomatoes, garlic, and cilantro.
Pretzel	On the street, these are big warm salty affairs that can stave off hunger in a pinch. They're 100% vegan.
Seitan	Gluten which has been boiled in a ginger-tamari broth.
Soy cheese	Soy milk processed to approximate the consistency and flavor of cheese. It almost always contains casein, a milk protein, so check to make sure it's vegan. (Soymage and Tofutti are typical brands of vegan cheese.)
Squash	A sweet autumn vegetable that comes in many types; pumpkin is one.
Tempeh	Fermented soybeans pressed into cakes, more flavorful than tofu.
Tempura	Vegetables dipped in batter and deep-fried. Ask about eggs in the batter.
Tofu	Tofu is to soy milk as cheese is to cow's milk. Relatively bland, it soaks up the flavors of whatever it's cooked in.
Zucchini	Courgette.

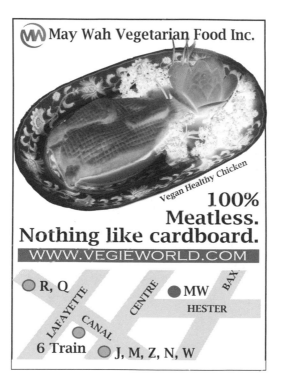

CRUELTY-FREE SHOES

Until recently, it was scandalous that in New York, one of the world's great pedestrian cities, there were no shops that specialized in selling vegetarian shoes. But now with the advent of shops like Moo Shoes and 99X, you can buy non-leather shoes that are durable, breathable, and good-looking.

MOOSHOES   78 Orchard Street
                                      bet. Stanton/ Rivington
Shoes, belts, and wallets all made by companies that make only leather-free goods.
www.mooshoes.com • 856-598-3426

99X   84 East 10th Street
Has a large vegan/vegetarian shoe section   bet. 3rd/ 4th Avenues
www. 99Xnyc.com • 212-460-8599

NY ARTIFICIAL   223 West 10th Street
                                      off Bleecker Street
NYA BLUE   13 8th Avenue
                                      at West 12th Street
NYA GREEN   13 8th Avenue
                                      at West 12th Street
Shoes, jewelry, accessories, handbags , apparel, and makeup.
www. nyartificial.com • 646-340-0442 • 646-340-0813

PAYLESS SHOE SOURCE   9 NYC locations; check phone book
Inexpensive, leather-look plastic shoes that last about 6 months.

STELLA McCARTNEY   429 West 14th Street
Non-leather shoes, accessories and clothing.
www.stellamccarney.com • 212-255-1556

MAIL ORDER

BLACKWELL'S ORGANIC VEGAN GELATO

9 Catherine Street, Unit D
Red Bank, NJ 07701
732-229-8899
www. blackwellsorganic.com

Vegan organic gelato and sorbetto available for shipment anywhere in the continental USA using FEDEX and dry ice.

PANGEA VEGAN PRODUCTS

283 Lewis Avenue
Rockville, MD 20851
1-800-340-1200
www.veganstore.com

A wide selection of dress shoes, casual shoes, hiking boots, athletic shoes and sandals. They also offer stylish faux leather coats, belts, wallets and bags.

USED RUBBER USA

597 Haight Street
San Francisco, CA 94117
415-626-7855
www.usedrubberusa.com

Wallets, bags, backpacks, dayplanners and address books made from recycled inner tubes.

HEARTLAND PRODUCTS, LTD.

Box 250
Dakota City, IA 50529
515-332-3087

Vegetarian footwear imported from England.

VEGETARIAN SHOES
British vegetarian shoes.

12 Gardner Street, Brighton, BN1
1UP, England
.0273-691913.

F & O ALTERNATIVE PET PRODUCTS
Vegan pet foods for dogs and cats.

11252 Fremont Avenue
Seattle, WA 98133
877-378-9056
www. vegancats.com

WHY VEGANISM?

Vegetarians avoid meat because of the animal suffering, negative health effects, and environmental damage involved in "eating carcasses," as Leo Tolstoy put it. Vegans carry these reasons to their logical conclusion and avoid using all animal products, to the extent possible.

Cruelty

Milk and eggs are taken from animals kept in horrific conditions on factory farms. Hens are packed into cages so small they would peck each other to death if their beaks hadn't been cut off by a hot knife; these cages are jammed into buildings housing as many as 80,000 birds. After a few exhausting years of laying eggs over conveyor belts with fluorescent lights on 18 hours a day, spent hens are turned into soup. In cows, as in women, there is a connection between lactation and pregnancy: cows only give milk after giving birth. Therefore cows are artificially inseminated every year and their calves are taken away to be slaughtered for pet food or raised for veal in confining crates. Cows are injected with hormones to increase their milk output, tranquilizers to calm them down and antibiotics to keep them from succumbing to the diseases they contract from the unhealthy conditions in which they are kept. After five or six years of this treatment they are slaughtered. (The natural lifespan of a cow is 20 years.)

Health

Eggs are high in cholesterol, which contributes to heart disease, the leading killer in the United States. Milk products such as whole milk, cheese and yogurt are high in cholesterol and saturated fat, which has been linked to heart disease and cancer. Even non-fat milk products can be harmful: recent studies have linked milk consumption to cataracts and a diet high in animal protein to osteoporosis; while the Recommended Dietary Allowance of protein (for men) is 63 grams, vegetarian men consume an average of 103 grams. Intolerance of milk is the most common food allergy, leading to flatulence and respiratory and skin problems. The U.S. Department of Agriculture estimates that 50% of the dairy cattle in the herds along Mexico's northern border—whose milk is sold in the U.S.—are infected with tuberculosis. And everything the cow eats, from antibiotics to pesticide-laden grain, winds up in her milk. The American Medical Association states that a vegan diet provides all required nutrients, including calcium, iron, and vitamin B-12. Olympic gold medalist Carl Lewis is a vegan—need we say more?

Environment

Animals are kept in such concentrations in factory farms or feedlots that tons of their wastes, laden with pesticide and chemical residue, become a hazard. Livestock production accounts for a staggering 50 percent of America's fresh water use. The runoff from cleaning stalls is contaminated and pollutes acquifers and rivers. Eighty percent of the herbicides used in the U.S. are sprayed on soybeans and corn, most of which are fed to livestock. Livestock raising is the primary cause of topsoil erosion in the United States, but that doesn't stop the U.S. government from spending $13 billion on price supports for milk. 64 percent of U.S. agricultural land is used for livestock feed. Shouldn't we eat the grain and leave the cow's secretions for her calf?

FOR MORE INFORMATION

ANIMALS, HEALTH, AND THE ENVIRONMENT

Farm Animal Reform Movement,10101 Ashburton Lane, Bethesda, MD 20817; ((888) **FARM-USA:** www. FARMUSA.org
Farm Sanctuary-Organization for the Rescue and Protection of Farm Animals, PO Box 150, Watkins Glen, NY 14891; ☎ (607) 583-2225
United Poultry Concerns, PO Box 150, Machipongo, VA 23405-0150, ☎ (757) 678-7875
Society & Animals Forum, PO Box 1297. Washington Grove, MD. 20880-1297. ☎ (301) 963-4751
Animal People, PO Box 960. Clinton, Washington, 98236-0960, MD. 20880-1297, ☎ (360) 579-2505
People for the Ethical Treatment of Animals, 501 Front Street, Norfolk, VA 23510; ☎ (757) 622-PETA
Friends of Animals 1841 Broadway, #812 , New York, NY 10023, ☎ (212) 247-8120
Animal Legal Defense Fund, 127 Fourth Street, Petaluma, CA 94952, ☎ (707) 769-7771
North American Vegetarian Society, PO Box 72, Dolgeville, NY 13329, ☎ (518) 568-7970
New York City Vegetarians, ☎ (718) 805-4260 Les Judd, or celiaveg@aol.com
Viva Vegie Society, home of the New York Vegetarian Center ☎212-242-0011.
American Vegan Society, 56 Dinshah Lane, PO Box 360, Malaga, NJ 08328, ☎ (856) 694-2887
Green Business in the Five Boroughs: 474 West 238th Street, #6, Bronx NY 10453, ☎ (718) 530-5074
Institute for Integrative Nutrition, 3 East 28th Street, 12th floor, NYC, NY 10016☎ (212) 730-5433. Offers natural cooking classes with no animal products.
Institute for Food and Health and The Natural Gourmet School, 48 West 21st St., 2nd Floor, ☎ (212) 645-5170. Natural cooking classes and a $20 Friday night vegan feast.
Earth Save New York, PO Box 96, NY, NY 10108, ☎ (212) 696-7986
Earth Save Long Island, PO Box 1313, Huntington, NY 11743, ☎ (800) 362-3648.

VEGAN DELIGHTS

Vegan Treats-Vegan Cakes and Pies ☎ (484) 239 8726; www. vegantreats.com
Vegethus Restaurante Best Vegan Satvic Homestyle Cuisine in South America, ☎ (11) 5539-3635, www. nutriveg.com.br
Vegan Chocolate Decadence, ☎ (800) 324-5018
Vegan Dried Fruits-Rainforest Delights, ☎ (626) 284-8001
Vegan Soaps,☎(877) 833-SOAP
Vegan Parmesan, Parma, ☎ (541) 665-0346
Vegan Organic Produce Home Delivery Service-Urban Organic, ☎ (718) 499-4321
Vegan Organic Cookies and Brownies-Allison's Gourmet, ☎ (800) 361-8292

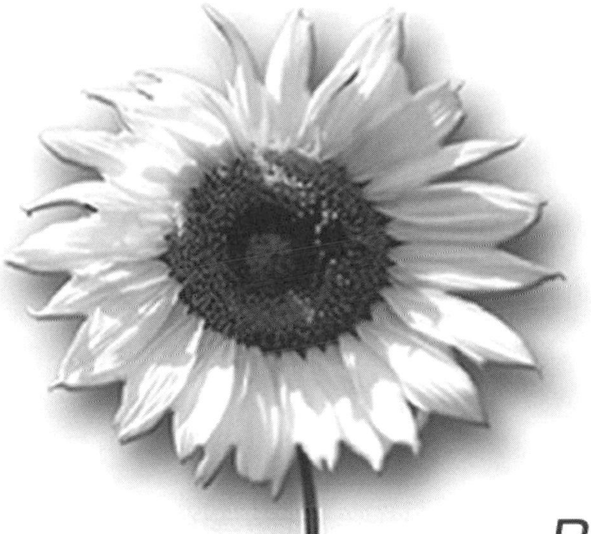

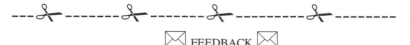

✉ FEEDBACK ✉

Please write to let us know how we can improve the next edition of The Vegan Guide to New York City. Tell us about new restaurants, changes, closings, great meals, whatever you like.

_____

_____

_____

_____

_____

_____

Your address: _____

_____

_____

_____

Additional copies.

For additional copies of *The Vegan Guide to New York City,* send $9.95 plus $1.50 postage each to:

Rynn Berry, 159 Eastern Parkway, Suite 2H, Brooklyn, NY 11238. tele/fax: (718) 622-8002. Email: berrynn@att.net. Web: vegsource.com/berry.

ALSO AVAILABLE: Rynn Berry's other bestselling books:
• *Famous Vegetarians* and *Their Favorite Recipes* @ $15.95 plus $3.00 postage.
• *Food for the Gods: Vegetarianism and the World's Religions* @ $19.95 plus $3.00 postage.
• *Hitler: Neither Vegetarian Nor Animal Lover* @ $10.95 plus $2.00 postage.
•*The New Vegetarians* @ $10.95 plus $2.00 postage

For copies of:
The Vegan Passport @ $5.00;Vegetarian London @ $10.00;
Vegetarian Britain @ $13.50; Vegetarian France @ $12.00;
Vegetarian Europe @ $13.50; send the designated amount, plus $2.00 postage, to Attention: Freya Dinshah, The American Vegan Society, 56 Dinshah Lane, PO Box 360, Malaga, NJ 08328 USA.

Notes

Notes

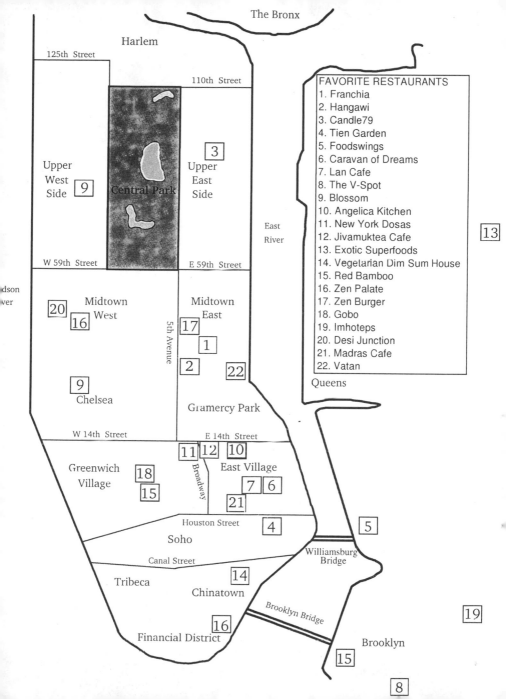

The Bronx

Harlem

125th Street

110th Street

Upper West Side [9]

Central Park

Upper East Side [3]

East River

W 59th Street

E 59th Street

FAVORITE RESTAURANTS
1. Franchia
2. Hangawi
3. Candle79
4. Tien Garden
5. Foodswings
6. Caravan of Dreams
7. Lan Cafe
8. The V-Spot
9. Blossom
10. Angelica Kitchen
11. New York Dosas
12. Jivamuktea Cafe
13. Exotic Superfoods
14. Vegetarian Dim Sum House
15. Red Bamboo
16. Zen Palate
17. Zen Burger
18. Gobo
19. Imhoteps
20. Desi Junction
21. Madras Cafe
22. Vatan

[13]

Hudson River

[20] Midtown West [16]

Midtown East

5th Avenue

[17]
[1]
[2]
[22]

[9]
Chelsea

Gramercy Park

Queens

W 14th Street

E 14th Street

[11] [12] [10]

Greenwich Village

[18]
[15]

Broadway

East Village

[7] [6]
[21]

Houston Street

[4]

[5]

Soho

Williamsburg Bridge

Canal Street

Tribeca

[14]

Chinatown

Brooklyn Bridge

[19]

[16]
Financial District

Brooklyn

[15]

[8]

Living Foods in the Caribbean

www.annwigmore.org

1 and 2 Week Programs
in the Tropics
with Ocean Access

We Work With Nature